Xiao Ou Xue
Yan Feng Liu

Herbal Medicine and Acupuncture for Menopausal Symptoms

Hoda Azizi
Xiao Ou Xue
Yan Feng Liu

Herbal Medicine and Acupuncture for Menopausal Symptoms

Herbal medicine and Acupuncture for the management of menopause related symptoms

Scholar's Press

Impressum / Imprint
Bibliografische Information der Deutschen Nationalbibliothek: Die Deutsche Nationalbibliothek verzeichnet diese Publikation in der Deutschen Nationalbibliografie; detaillierte bibliografische Daten sind im Internet über http://dnb.d-nb.de abrufbar.

Bibliographic information published by the Deutsche Nationalbibliothek: The Deutsche Nationalbibliothek lists this publication in the Deutsche Nationalbibliografie; detailed bibliographic data are available in the Internet at http://dnb.d-nb.de.

Coverbild / Cover image: www.ingimage.com

Verlag / Publisher:
Scholar's Press
ist ein Imprint der / is a trademark of
OmniScriptum GmbH & Co. KG
Heinrich-Böcking-Str. 6-8, 66121 Saarbrücken, Deutschland / Germany
Email: info@scholars-press.com

Herstellung: siehe letzte Seite /
Printed at: see last page
ISBN: 978-3-639-51511-4

Zugl. / Approved by: Beijing, Beijing University of Chinese Medicine, 2009

Contents

Abbreviations:

- ACU — Acupuncture
- CAM — Complementary and Alternative Medicine
- E2 — Estradiol
- EA — Electro Acupuncture
- FMP — Final Menstrual Period
- FSH — Follicle Stimulating Hormone
- HERS — Heart and Estrogen-progestin Replacement Study
- HRT — Hormone Replacement Therapy
- HT — Hormone Therapy
- KBW — Kun Bao Wan
- KI — Kupperman Index
- LH — Luteinizing Hormone
- MRS — Menopause Related Symptoms
- NS — Number of Symptoms
- QOL — Quality Of Life
- SSC……………………Symptom Severity Score
- STRAW — Stages of Reproductive Aging Workshop
- VMS — Vasomotor Symptoms
- WHI — Women's Health Initiative

Abstract

Abstract (English):

Back ground: Menopause Related Symptoms affect women's mid-life quality of life and impose immense psychological and socioeconomic burden on women's life. Current conventional therapy is Hormone Therapy. Concerns about the safety of Estrogen-based hormone replacement therapy have led to demand for other options like CAM; however, the efficacy and adverse effects of non hormonal therapies are unclear.

Material and Methods: In this clinical trial, we divided 57 patients with MRS (including peri and post menopause) to three treatment groups: Chinese herbal formula (Kun Bao Wan 500 gr BID, n=22), Acupuncture + Kun Bao Wan (Kun Bao Wan 500 gr BID + 10 sessions of acupuncture; kidney tonifying protocol, n=20), and Hormone therapy (n=15). The duration of treatment was 8 weeks for every patient. Outcome measures were Kupperman Index, FSH, E2, LH and number of symptoms. This study was enrolled in two university affiliated hospitals in the city of Beijing; Dongzhimen Hospital and Beijing University People Hospital. Data was analyzed with ANOVA, paired and independent sample t-test and chi-square test. Level of significance was 0.05.

Results: KBW, ACU+KBW and HT significantly decreased Kupperman Index of patients ($P<0.001$). Mean and Standard Deviation of KI decrease was 8.59 ± 6.005 in KBW group, 14.55 ± 8.46 in ACU+KBW group and 11.13 ± 5.80 in HT group which were significantly different according to ANOVA test ($P= 0.02$). Tukey test showed that the difference was due to the significantly better effect of ACU + KBW than KBW. There was no significant difference neither between the effect of KBW and HT nor ACU+KBW and HT. Moreover, the effect of three treatments on lowering the severity score of hot flash was not significantly different.
Each of three treatment groups decreased patients' number of symptoms significantly ($p<0.05$) but the difference between treatment groups was not significant.
ACU+KBW and HT significantly decreased the level of FSH ($P<0.05$). KBW and HT significantly decreased the level of LH ($P<0.05$). KBW didn't make a significant decrease in the Level of FSH in patients. ACU+KBW didn't make a significant decrease in the Level of LH in patients. The three treatments didn't make any significant increase in the level of E2.
We also compared the effects of 3 treatments between perimenopause and postmenopause patients. In Perimenopause patients there was no significant difference between three treatments' effect on KI ($P>0.05$); but in Post menopause patients there was a significant difference between KBW and ACU+KBW ($P=0.01$); also KBW and HT ($P=0.027$).
There was a correlation between response to the treatment by lowering KI and severity of Hot flash ($r=-0.46$, $p<0.001$), Insomnia ($r=-0.27$, $p=0.03$), weakness ($r= -0.38$, $p=0.003$), palpitation ($r=-0.56$, $p<0.001$) and having "5 zone hot sensations" before the treatment. This study suggests these symptoms to be prognostic factors for response to the treatment.

Conclusion: Kun Bao Wan and acupuncture as two Traditional Chinese Medicine treatments, significantly decreased the symptoms of women with MRS; even acupuncture + KBW was as effective as conventional hormone therapy in decreasing the symptoms and in changing the hormonal levels.

Key words: Menopause, Acupuncture, Kun Bao Wan, Hormone therapy, Chinese Medicine

Abstract (Chinese):

摘　要

背景：

随绝经而出现的一系列症状对女性生活有着很大影响，给她们精神和经济上带来极大负担。对这些症状的常规治疗为激素疗法，因考虑雌激素替代疗法的安全性问题，故我们试图寻找更理想的治疗方法，比如 CAM。但非激素疗法的疗效和副作用还有待进一步研究。

资料和方法：

在临床研究中，我们把 57 名病人（包括围绝经期和绝经 1 年后病人）分为 3 组：坤宝丸组（n=22），针刺+坤宝丸组（n=20）和激素疗法组（n=15）。每组疗程均为 8 周，针刺+坤宝丸组的病人服用坤宝丸，同时接受 10 次针刺治疗。通过比较病人治疗前后的库帕曼指数，FSH, LH, E2 和症状的变化来评价各组治疗方法。此项研究在北京两所大学的附属医院进行：东直门医院和北京大学人民医院。数据分析采用方差分析，配对和独立样本 t-检验以及卡方检验。

结果：

坤宝丸组，针刺+坤宝丸组和激素疗法组都显著降低病人的库帕曼指数($P<0.001$)。库帕曼指数的平均值和标准差为：坤宝丸组 8.59 ± 6.005，坤宝丸+针刺组 14.55 ± 8.46，激素疗法组 11.13 ± 5.80，根据方差分析($P= 0.02$)有显著性差异。经图基检验（Tukey test），差异来源于针刺+坤宝丸组显著优于坤宝丸组。坤宝丸组和激素疗法组，以及针刺+坤宝丸组和激素疗法组之间没有显著差异。此外，三组疗法在降低病人潮热症状的评分中无显著性差异。

每组疗法对降低病人的症状均有显著疗效($P<0.05$)，但各组间无显著性差异。

针刺+坤宝丸组和激素疗法组显著降低 FSH 水平($P<0.05$)。坤宝丸组和激素疗法组显著降低 LH 水平($P<0.05$)。坤宝丸组在降低 FSH 水平上无显著差异。针刺+坤宝丸组在降低 LH 水平上无显著差异。三组在升高 E2 水平上无显著差异。

我们还比较了三组疗法分别对围绝经期和绝经 1 年后病人的结果。三组疗法对降低围绝经期病人的库帕曼指数无显著差异($P>0.05$)；但是在绝经 1 年后病人中，坤宝丸组和针刺+坤宝丸组之间有显著差异(P=0.01)；坤宝丸组和激素疗法组之间有显著差异(P=0.027)。

库帕曼指数降低和以下症状改善之间显示有相关性：潮热(r=-0.46, p<0.001),失眠(r=-0.27, p=0.03),疲劳(r= -0.38, p=0.003),心悸 (r=-0.56, p<0.001)，以及治疗前的“五心烦热”。研究发现这些症状的减轻预示着疗效的显著。

结论：

坤宝丸和针刺作为两项传统中医疗法，对减轻随绝经而出现的一系列症状上有显著疗效；针刺+坤宝丸在减轻症状和改变激素水平上与常规激素疗法同样有效。

关键词： 绝经，针刺，坤宝丸，激素疗法，中医

Abstract (Persian):

مقدمه: شکايات وابسته به منوپوز به طور شايعي کيفيت زندگي خانم هاي ميانسال را تحت تاثير قرار مي دهند و بار جسمي، رواني، اجتماعي و اقتصادي زيادي بر خانم هاي ين محدوده سني اعمال مي کنند. درمان رايج طبي در حال حاضر درمان هورموني است. نگراني هايي که به دنبال مطالعات درباره ايمني درمانهاي هورموني حاوي استروژن به وجود آمد، منجر به افزايش درخواست ها براي درمانهاي جايگزين و مکمل شد، هر چند کارايي و عوارض جانبي درمانهاي غير هورموني هنوز مشخص نيست.

مواد و روشها: در اين کارآزمايي باليني، ۵۷ بيمار مبتلا به شکايات وابسته به منوپوز اعم از خانم هاي دوره حول و حوش يائسگي و خانم هاي يائسه به طور تصادفي به سه گروه تقسيم شدند: گروه درمان با فرمولاسيون گياهي KBW(n=22)، گروه درمان با طب سوزني+ فرمولاسيون گياهي KBW (n=20) و گروه هورمون درماني(n=15). مدت درمان ۸ هفته بود. گروه دوم علاوه بر درمان گياهي ۱۰ جلسه تحت درمان با طب سوزني قرار گرفتند. پاسخ درماني بر اساس تغييرات در اندکس کوپرمن، سطح هورمونهاي FSH، LH و E2 و تعداد علايم بيمار قبل و بعد از درمان مورد ارزيابي قرار گرفت. مطالعه در دو مرکز دانشگاهي بيمارستان دنگ جي من و بيمارستان خلق در شهر پکن کشور چين به انجام رسيد. تحليل داده ها با استفاده از تست هاي آماري ANOVA ، paired and independent sample t-test و chi-square انجام شد و۰,۰۵ به عنوان سطح معناداري در نظر گرفته شد.

نتايج: KBW ، "طب سوزني+KBW" و هورمون درماني به طور معني داري اندکس کوپرمن بيماران را پايين آوردند (P<0.001). ميانگين و SD کاهش اندکس کوپرمن در گروه KBW 8.59±6.005، در گروه "طب سوزني+KBW" 14.55±8.46 و در گروه هورمون درماني 11.13±5.80 بود که بر اساس تست ANOVA به طور معني داري متفاوت بودند (P= 0.02).بر اساس تست توکي اين تفاوت مربوط به برتري معني دار گروه "طب سوزني+KBW" نسبت به گروه KBW بود اما بين گروه هورمون درماني با KBW و "طب سوزني+KBW" تفاوت معني داري وجود نداشت. اثر سه گروه بر کاهش شدت حملات گرگرفتگي يکسان بود. هر سه درمان به طور معني داري تعداد علايم بيماران را کاهش دادند(p<0.05) و اختلاف معني داري با هم نداشتند. "طب سوزني+KBW" و هورمون درماني به طور معني داري سطح FSH را کاهش دادند (P<0.05) اما KBW اثر معنا داري در کاهش FSH ايجاد نکرد. هيچ يک از سه درمان افزايش معني داري در سطح E2 ايجاد نکردند. KBW و هورمون درماني سطح LH را به طور معني داري کاهش دادند.

بين کاهش اندکس کوپرمن بيماران و شدت گرگرفتگي، بيخوابي، ضعف و خستگي، تپش قلب و داشتن علامت احساس داغي در ۵ ناحيه (مربوط به نشانه شناسي طب چيني) قبل از درمان همبستگي يافت شد بنابر اين اين مطالعه، علايم فوق الذکر را به عنوان فاکتورهاي پروگنوستيک پاسخ به درمان معرفي مي کند.

نتيجه گيري: طب سوزني و فرمولاسيون گياهي Kun Bao Wan به عنوان دو درمان طب چيني در درمان شکايات مربوط به منوپوز به طور معني داري موثر هستند.

کليد واژه ها: Menopause ، Acupuncture، Kun Bao Wan، Hormone therapy، Chinese Medicine

Chapter One

Introduction

1-1 Definition:

Menopause is a natural process that occurs in women's lives as part of normal aging. Many women go through the menopausal transition with few or no symptoms, while some have significant or even disabling symptoms. Menopause is defined by the World Health Organization and the Stages of Reproductive Aging Workshop (STRAW) working group as the permanent cessation of menstrual periods that occurs naturally or is induced by surgery, chemotherapy, or radiation. Natural menopause is recognized after 12 consecutive months without menstrual periods that are not associated with a physiologic (e.g., lactation) or pathologic cause. Menopausal transition often begins with variations in length of the menstrual cycle. The hormonal changes during the menopausal transition can span several years.

The following three periods or intervals were defined by experts at the STRAW working group in 2001:

1. *Reproductive stage*: From menarche (first menstrual period) to the beginning of the perimenopause (when cycles become variable).

2. *Menopausal transition*: The time of an increase in follicle-stimulating hormone and increased variability in cycle length, 2 skipped menstrual cycles with 60 or more days of amenorrhea (absence of menstruation), or both. The menopausal transition concludes with the final menstrual period (FMP) and the beginning of postmenopause.

3. *Postmenopause*: Begins at the time of the FMP, although it is not recognized until after 12 months of amenorrhea. [1]

FIGURE Schematic of the Menopausal Transition

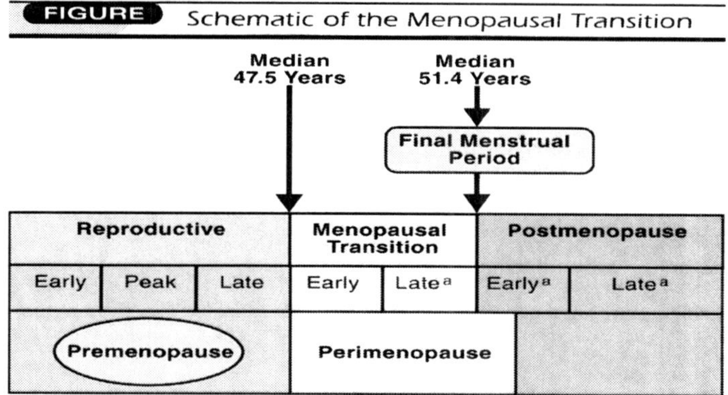

In this text, we use the term *menopausal transition* to mean the time from the late reproductive stage and entry into postmenopause. The term *perimenopause* is defined as the period immediately prior to menopause (when the biological and

clinical features of approaching menopause begin) and the first year after menopause. Thus, perimenopause includes the menopausal transition and overlaps the first 12 months of postmenopause.
Menopause is a term that is often used to describe perimenopause or the menopausal transition when in fact it refers to a specific point in time. Menopause does not technically occur until 12 months after the last menstrual period.

When menopause occurs naturally, it generally affects women aged 40 to 58 years (median onset of menopausal transition: 47.5 years), although premature menopause (i.e., menopause that occurs in women aged < 40 years) may occur.

The menopause-related symptoms include irregular menstrual periods, vasomotor symptoms (VMS) (i.e., hot flashes [rapid onset of intense heat sensation, sweating, and flushing lasting approximately 5-10 minutes], night sweats), sleep disturbances, vulvovaginal atrophy (e.g., dryness, itching, burning), sexual dysfunction, mood disturbances (depression, anxiety, and irritability), and somatic symptoms (back pain, tiredness, and stiff or painful joints). [1],[2],[3]
Of these, VMS are the most bothersome and are the main focus of menopausal treatment guidelines. [4]

Because women age as they progress from premenopause to postmenopause, it is difficult to determine which symptoms occurring during this time are due to ovarian aging specifically and which are due to general aging and/or life changes commonly experienced in midlife. NIH Consens State described these symptoms and their relation to menopause by the following discussion.

Vasomotor Symptoms (Hot Flashes and Night Sweats):
The vasomotor symptoms of hot flashes—sudden sensations of intense heat with sweating and flushing typically lasting 5 to 10 minutes—and night sweats are reported with high frequency in perimenopausal women. There is strong evidence from both longitudinal and cross-sectional observational studies that the menopausal transition causes vasomotor symptoms. Hot flashes rarely occur before women enter the perimenopausal transition and occur in a higher percentage of women in the later phases of the menopausal transition. They also occur with a higher frequency and greater severity in younger women who undergo a sudden onset of menopause due to surgical removal of their ovaries or medical conditions or treatments that decrease the ability of ovaries to produce hormones. Further evidence supporting this association is provided by the large number of good-quality interventional clinical trials demonstrating improvement of vasomotor symptoms with estrogen treatment.

Vaginal Dryness and Painful Intercourse
Vaginal dryness, often leading to painful intercourse (dyspareunia), is reported by many perimenopausal and postmenopausal women. Evidence from observational

studies that menopause causes vaginal dryness is strong. The percentage of women experiencing vaginal dryness increases throughout the menopausal transition and persists indefinitely in some women. Increases in vaginal dryness correlate well with the onset of the menopausal transition. Microscopic examination of vaginal cells obtained from postmenopausal women reporting vaginal dryness shows changes consistent with low estrogen levels. Furthermore, treatment of vaginal dryness with estrogen (either vaginal or systemic) results in relief of symptoms, including menopause-associated dyspareunia, for most women.

Sleep Disturbance

Sleep disturbances are common and increase with age in both men and women across the lifespan for a variety of reasons. There is moderate evidence from longitudinal cohort and cross-sectional observational studies that menopause is the cause of such disturbances in some women. The role of vasomotor symptoms in sleep disturbances remains unclear.

Mood Symptoms

From observational studies, there is limited evidence that ovarian changes associated with menopause might be a cause of depression, anxiety, and/or irritability. History of prior depression, life stress, and general health are the major predictors of mood symptoms during midlife. Because of the multiple potential causes of mood changes and the relatively high proportion of women reporting one or more of these symptoms, it is difficult to establish whether menopause causes any increase in the prevalence of mood symptoms during the perimenopausal years. The evidence from estrogen treatment trials is mixed, with only weak evidence of improvement in depression or anxiety relative to placebo for a small subset of moderately or highly symptomatic women treated with estrogens. [1] A recent study published in *Menopause* 2009 showed that changes in Estradiol and, to a lesser extent, in FSH levels are associated with an increased risk of depressive symptoms in postmenopausal women. These results further support a role for **fluctuating** rather than absolute hormone levels in depression in later life. [5]

Cognitive Disturbances

There is insufficient information to conclude that there is any causal relationship between the menopausal transition and difficulty thinking, forgetfulness, or other cognitive disturbances. Existing studies are inadequate for separating aging effects from the effects of menopause.

Somatic Symptoms

The majority of studies showed no association between the prevalence of somatic symptoms, including back pain, tiredness, and stiff or painful joints, and menopausal status.

Urinary Incontinence

In a small number of longitudinal and cross-sectional studies that considered associations between menopausal status and urinary incontinence, results are mixed. Current results are inadequate to demonstrate a causal relationship.

Uterine Bleeding Problems
The menopausal transition is, by definition, associated with alteration in menstrual cycles. In addition, menorrhagia (excessive bleeding) has frequently been reported by perimenopausal women. There are no adequate long-term studies examining menorrhagia during the menopausal transition. Any such studies would need to account for the presence of fibroids and other uterine conditions.

Sexual Dysfunction
Two components of sexual dysfunction during the menopausal transition have been identified: painful intercourse resulting from vaginal atrophy and dryness, as discussed earlier, and changes in libido, arousal, and other aspects of sexuality. These latter three changes are strongly associated with age-related factors, such as changes in personal relationships, stressors, and socioeconomic conditions. Their association with menopausal hormone changes has not been established definitively. [1]

1-2 Epidemiological aspects of Menopause and Menopause Related symptoms:

Age of onset:
Menopausal symptoms vary among women at each stage of the menopausal transition and also vary for each woman over time as she goes through these stages. In the United States, most women experience menopause between 40 and 58 years of age, with a median age of 52 years. Factors associated with earlier menopause include lower body weight, menstrual length, nulliparity, smoking, never-use of oral contraceptives, lower socioeconomic status, and race or ethnicity. Higher body weight is associated with later onset of menopause.
Some women who transit menopause have no symptoms at all, but most experience some symptoms, often beginning several years before the FMP. Understanding the natural history of menopausal symptoms requires long-term data on numerous women from diverse backgrounds. To date, most longitudinal studies have followed women for 2 to 8 years, which is not long enough to define the natural history of menopausal symptoms during the menopausal transition and into later life.
Menopausal symptoms are higher in early and late perimenopause than in pre- or postmenopause, except vaginal dryness (whose prevalence continues to rise across these stages).

Prevalence of Menopause Related symptoms:
- Vasomotor Symptoms (Hot Flashes and Night Sweats):

The estimates of prevalence of vasomotor symptoms vary from 14 to 51 percent in premenopause, from 35 to 50 percent in perimenopause, and from 30 to 80 percent in postmenopause. [1] A recent study in 2008 states that 75% of women aged over 50 years experience the most bothersome symptoms of menopause which are vasomotor symptoms (VMS), such as hot flashes and night sweats. [4] High body mass index and younger age of onset of menopause are associated with more vasomotor symptoms. After the WHI study results were published, many women in clinical settings stopped hormone therapy. In one study, among women who had discontinued hormonal therapy, 25 percent resumed therapy because of symptoms. This suggests that there may be a subgroup of women for whom symptoms are so severe that they may be willing to accept some increased risk for long-term complications.

- Vaginal Dryness and Painful Intercourse:

Vaginal dryness becomes increasingly more common throughout the menopausal transition. Estimates of the prevalence of vaginal dryness vary from 4 to 22 percent in premenopause, from 7 to 39 percent in perimenopause, and from 17 to 30 percent in postmenopause.

- Sleep Disturbance:

The prevalence of sleep disturbance varies from 16 to 42 percent in premenopause, from 39 to 47 percent in perimenopause, and from 35 to 60 percent in postmenopause.

- Mood Symptoms:

In different studies, the prevalence of mood symptoms varied from 8 to 37 percent in the premenopause, from 11 to 21 percent in perimenopause, and from 8 to 38 percent in postmenopause (natural or surgical).

- Other Symptoms:

Estimates of the prevalence of urinary symptoms vary from 10 to 36 percent in premenopause, from 17 to 39 percent in perimenopause, and from 15 to 36 percent in postmenopause (natural or surgical).

No association seems to exist for increased physical symptoms or cognitive problems during the menopausal transition.

Women in the age range of menopause experience an increase in sexual dysfunction (changes in libido, arousal and other aspects of sexuality). Although an association between sexual dysfunction and vaginal dryness is plausible, studies of the association were not available.

Overall, the natural history of menopausal symptoms may differ among racial or ethnic groups and for women with surgically induced menopause. [1]

Effect of VMS on the Quality of life:

The impact of VMS has gained in importance as the lifespan of women has increased throughout the world since women can expect to spend a significant portion of their lives after menopause. This period should be a highly productive time for women, and maintaining functional ability and a good QOL is of utmost importance. VMS can have a significant negative impact on QOL in younger and older women, contributing to physical as well as psychosocial impairment. [6] Becoming flushed and sweating profusely in a social or work-related situation may cause extreme anxiety for many women and lead to social isolation. [7]

According to a recent study by "Worldwide Epidemiology" Hot flashes affected work (46.0%), social activities (44.4%), leisure activities (47.6%), sleep (82.0%), mood (68.6%), concentration (69.0%), sexual activity (40.9%), total energy level (63.3%) and overall quality of life (69.3%). [8]

Burden of disease (physical, psychosocial, financial):
VMS are the leading reason why women seek medical attention for menopause.
The top 4 reasons for seeking medical attention identified in a 2002 Gallup poll of menopausal women were hot flashes (70%), night sweats (68%), mood disturbances (50%), and sleep disturbances (49%). [6] These data are supported by results of a more recent poll, which showed that 60% of peri- and postmenopausal women sought care for their menopausal symptoms. [9]
On average, most women experience VMS for 6 months to 2 years; however, approximately 10% of women report experiencing VMS for 10 or more years. [6],[10]
Worldwide, between 50% and 85% of women (approximately 360 million) older than 45 years of age experience hot flushes [11]
According to U.S. census data, there are more than 48 million American women aged over 50 years, and nearly 60 million women aged 45 years and over. [12]
Considering the fact that all these women will go through menopause, 75% of them will experience VMS [6], and 60% of them will seek medical attention for their symptoms, [9] it isn't surprising that the financial burden of VMS is immense. Direct costs incurred by women with menopause-associated VMS include initial and follow-up physician office visits and telephone calls, which may include visits to specialists (e.g., psychologist, psychiatrist, neurologist), as well as primary care physicians or gynecologists, prescription, and over-the-counter (OTC) medications, dietary supplements, and laboratory tests[6]. Indirect costs include loss of productivity at home or at work, hygiene-related supplies, increased energy usage for air conditioning and laundry, and management of treatment-related adverse events. One cost-effectiveness comparison estimated the yearly cost of VMS management to average $681 to $848 per patient per year. [13]

1-3 Pathophysiology and treatment of menopause Related symptoms (MRS) in Conventional Medicine:

1-3-1 Pathophysiology of MRS:

There is currently no consensus on the pathophysiology of menopause associated VMS; however, many hypotheses have been proposed.
In Western Medicine, the exact pathophysiology of the hot flushes is still unknown but it could be related to an alteration in the set point temperature in the hypothalamus. [14] Both withdrawal and activation of endogenous opioids, e.g. Beta endorphin, have been suggested as underlying mechanisms; however, current evidence is insufficient because of lack of studies with appropriate design. Hot flushes were proposed to be hypothalamic thermoregulatory events originating from increased brain norepinephrine activity, due to decreased activity of hypothalamic opioids, which in turn is caused by estrogen withdrawal. [15], [16]

This was supported by the finding that hot flushes diminished with pharmacotherapy that increased opioid concentrations. [17] Nonetheless, opioid activation was also suspected because people receiving Chlorpropamide flush after drinking alcohol. [18] Further, it was hypothesized that estrogen withdrawal could lead to reduction in the blood Serotonin (5-HT) level and consequently to an up-regulation of 5-HT_{2A} receptors. The activation of 5-HT_{2A} receptors might disturb the hypothalamic set point temperature, which activates autonomic reactions to cool down the body, such as vasodilatation causing increased skin temperature and sweating. [19] It was shown that 5-HT level was restored to normal after treatment with estrogen in women with spontaneous and surgical menopause. [20],[21] Narrowing of the thermoregulatory threshold between sweating and shivering in the hypothalamus is a proposed mechanism for hot flashes. [22] This narrowing is thought to be caused by Changes in the levels of circulating serotonin (decreasing concentration), norepinephrine (increasing concentration), or estrogen (decreasing concentration). [2], [10] The postmenopausal decline in ovarian estradiol production results in diminished negative-feedback effects on the anterior pituitary, leading to a compensatory increase in the secretion of luteinizing hormone from the pituitary, a process regulated by gonadotropin-releasing hormone in the hypothalamus. [23] Pulsatile surges of gonadotropin-releasing hormone due to estrogen deficiency affect the hypothalamic neurons that control central thermoregulation centers. [24]

It has also been hypothesized that the ratios of the specific pes of estrogen (i.e., estradiol or estrone) may be better correlated with the occurrence of VMS than the overall circulating level of estrogen. [25] Estrone, which is much lower in potency than estradiol, is the most abundant circulating estrogen in postmenopausal women. In premenopausal women, estradiol is the more abundant estrogen. [23] Further, the occurrence of VMS has been found to correlate better with ***an acute decline*** in estrogen levels than with the actual measured levels of estrogen. [10] In addition to the impact of the ***change in the relative amounts of estradiol and estrone***, another hypothesized contributor to VMS is the ***actual function of the available circulating estrogen***. For example, the cytochrome p450 isoenzyme CYP1A1 is responsible for the hydroxylation of estrone and estradiol, forming hydroxyestrone (2HE). 2HE binds very weakly to the estrogen receptor. [25],[26]

The relative amounts of the more potent estradiol is also affected by 17βhydroxysteroid dehydrogenase (17HSD), the enzyme responsible for the bidirectional conversion of the less potent estrone and the more potent estradiol. [25], [26] Alterations in the estrogen receptors ERα and ERβ may also negatively affect the biologic activity of estrogen. [27] It has been shown in one study that single nucleotide polymorphisms (SNPs) in the genes encoding estrogen metabolizing enzymes (i.e., CYP1A1, CYP1B1, 17HSD) or ERs are associated with prevalence of VMS, and ***these polymorphisms correlate with ethnic differences in VMS prevalence*** noted previously. [25] Additional studies are needed to confirm these results and further clarify the pathophysiology of VMS.

1-3-2 Hormonal changes during perimenopause:

The menopausal transition is the stage in reproductive life commonly defined as commencing with the onset of menstrual irregularity. Classic studies of the endocrinology of the transition postulated the existence of inhibin in women to explain the observed increase in follicle-stimulating hormone (FSH) levels without a significant decrease in estradiol (E2). Descriptions were provided of cycle characteristics during the transition, emphasizing the unpredictability of the endocrine changes rather than the occurrence of an orderly and progressive decline in ovarian function. Women older than the age of 45 exhibited menstrual irregularity when the average number of primordial follicles per ovary decreased to approximately 100. Inhibin B is a major regulator of FSH secretion and a product of small antral follicles. Its levels respond to the early follicular phase increase and decrease in FSH. The age-related decrease in ovarian primordial follicle numbers, which is reflected in a decrease in the numbers of small antral follicles, leads to a decrease in inhibin B, which in turn leads to an increase in FSH, hypothesized to act as a stimulus to the maintenance of circulating E2 in the follicular phase until late in the transition. Concurrently, the concentrations of testosterone do not change significantly. Early follicular phase FSH levels in women reporting menstrual irregularity fluctuate markedly, with a more uniform increase in levels when no menses have occurred for at least 3 months. Anovulatory cycles occur at increased frequency in the last 30 months before final menses or menopause. In ovulatory cycles, FSH shows little, if any, increase, but anovulatory cycles are usually characterized by low levels of inhibin B, markedly increased levels of FSH, and low levels of E2. Thus, the heterogeneity of follicular phase FSH represents a mixture of ovulat ory and anovulatory cycles. Longitudinal data indicate that both ovulatory and anovulatory cycles occur after entry into both the early and late menopausal transition and that ovulatory cycles occur even after final menses. There is no endocrine marker of menopause, which may be primarily an endometrial event. Using the hormonal concentrations in ovulatory cycles observed in women in mid-reproductive age as controls and comparing such concentrations in late reproductive age women older than 45 either continuing to cycle regularly or having entered the early or late menopausal transition, a gradual increase in follicular phase FSH and E2 and a decrease in inhibin B were observed in ovulatory cycles. Anovulatory cycles showed markedly increased FSH with low E2 and inhibin B. No specific endocrine change was characteristic of either the early or late menopausal transition, confirming the observations of previous studies regarding the unpredictability of cycle characteristics and hormone changes with the approach of menopause. Antimullerian hormone correlates with follicle numbers and shows a large age-related decrease to reach undetectable levels at menopause. Thus, the marked decrease in follicle numbers during late reproductive age appears to predispose to erratic and unpredictable cycle characteristics, with normal ovulatory cycles continuing to occur episodically. There is no specific endocrine marker of the early or late transition, making measurements of FSH or E2 unreliable in attempting to stage an individual with regard to approaching menopause. [28]

1-3-3 Treatment of VMS in conventional medicine:

Current treatment of menopause-associated VMS is centered on a foundation of lifestyle changes in all women and Hormone Replacement Therapy in women with moderate-to-severe VMS.

These days, Women are increasingly encouraged to participate in making decisions about hormone therapy. However, the complexity and uncertainty of information about the treatment can make it difficult for women to make a decision, increasing their reliance on medical advice. [29]

Since Hormone Therapy was introduced 80 years ago, a steady flow of studies has produced evidence of both harmful and beneficial effects. The publication of the Heart and Estrogen-progestin Replacement Study (HERS) [30] and Women's Health Initiative (WHI) [31] study, both of which found adverse effects, has added to the confusion.

1-3-4 Benefits and risks of Hormone Therapy

A- Benefits:

The main reasons for prescribing hormone therapy are relief of menopausal symptoms and prevention or management of osteoporosis. Some evidence also exists that it may have a role in primary and secondary prevention of cardiovascular disease, prevention of colorectal cancer, and prevention of Alzheimer's disease.

Relief of menopausal symptom: Although women report that hormone therapy improves various menopausal symptoms, [32] randomised clinical trials have proved that it is effective for only vasomotor [33] and urogenital symptoms. [34] A "domino" effect may occur—for example, relieving hot flushes may improve sleep, which may improve mood. In addition, Estrogen has been found to improve quality of life in the short term. [35]

Prevention or management of osteoporosis: After the age of 35 years, men and women start to lose around 1% of bone mass each year. However, bone loss is accelerated during the first three to four years after the menopause. A third of women over the age of 50 years sustain a fracture, with osteopenia a major risk factor. [36]

Women with specific risk factors should be offered bone density screening (preferably dual x ray absorptiometry) and those with a low bone mass offered hormone replacement therapy or other anti-resorptive treatment. Follow up bone density measurements can be used to adjust the dose of hormone replacement therapy and ensure women maintain adequate bone mass. Randomised controlled trials have shown that hormone replacement therapy reduces bone loss at clinically relevant sites such as the spine (reduced by 50%) and neck of femur (by 30%). In addition, a review of randomised trials reported a significant reduction in fractures in women taking hormone replacement therapy. This effect, however, may be less in women older than 60. [37]

The WHI study was the first randomised controlled trial to show a reduction in hip fracture with hormone replacement therapy. [31]

Bone loss resumes within a year after stopping hormone replacement therapy, however, and bone turnover rises to the level of that in untreated women within three to six months. Non-hormonal therapies such as bisphosphonates and selective oestrogen receptor modulators are as effective as hormone replacement therapy for preventing fractures. These are a good treatment for women with low bone mineral density who do not have problematic hypo-oestrogenic symptoms, have contraindications to hormone replacement therapy, or do not wish to take it.

Royal College of Physicians guidance on risk factors for osteoporosis:

- Premature menopause (before the age of 40)
- Family history of osteoporosis
- Taken steroids for more than 6 months
- Premenopausal amenorrhea for more than 6 months (due to low body mass index or excessive exercise)
- Liver, thyroid, or renal disease
- History of excessive alcohol intake
- Taken gonadotrophin releasing hormone analogues for more than 6 months

Colorectal cancer

Observational studies have consistently suggested that Menopause Hormone Therapy (HT) reduces the risk of colorectal cancer. [38] The WHI study, however, was the first randomised controlled trial to confirmthis, reporting six fewer colorectal cancers each year in every 10 000 women taking hormone replacement therapy compared with the placebo group. [31] The mechanisms behind this reduction in colorectal cancer are not clear.

HT and Cardiovascular disease:

Cardiovascular disease rarely affects women before the menopause, strongly implicating oestrogen deficiency in the aetiology of the disease. Observational studies have reported that oestrogen decreases morbidity and mortality from coronary heart disease by 30-50%. [40] This benefit is reduced, however, by the addition of progestogens, which are needed to prevent endometrial disease. [41]. Indeed, the WHI and HERS double blind, randomised, placebo controlled trials have shown that continuous treatment with 0.625 mg of conjugated equine oestrogens plus 2.5 mg of medroxyprogesterone increases the risk of heart disease events by 29% (37 v 30 per 10 000 person years) and stroke by 41% (29 v 21 per 10 000 person years). [30], [31], [42]

B- Risks:

Hormone replacement therapy seems to be associated with an increased risk of breast cancer, myocardial infarction, cerebrovascular disease, and thromboembolic disease. [39]

HT and Thromboembolic disease:

Studies generally show an increased risk of deep vein thrombosis and pulmonary embolus in women taking hormone replacement therapy. [43], [44], [45]

The absolute risk in current users is small, with estimates of 16 and 23 excess cases per 100 000 women a year for all venous thromboembolism and 6 per 10 000 women a year for pulmonary embolism. Women taking hormone replacement therapy have twice the risk of venous thromboembolism compared with non-users. The increase in risk seems to be greater in the first year of use, with an odds ratio of 4.6 (95% confidence interval 2.5 to 8.4) during the first six months. Hormone replacement therapy may therefore be unmasking an underlying thrombophilic tendency. The risks of venous thromboembolism with hormone replacement therapy are likely to be greater in women with predisposing factors such as a family history of thromboembolic disease, severe varicose veins, obesity, surgery, trauma, or prolonged bed rest, and age is an important risk factor.

HT and Breast cancer:

A serious concern for women taking long term hormone replacement therapy is the reported increased risk of breast cancer. [46] The risk is higher with oestrogen-progestogen combinations than with oestrogen alone.

HT and Endometrial cancer:

The increased incidence of endometrial hyperplasia and endometrial cancer associated with unopposed hormone replacement therapy has been established since the 1970s. Progestogen decreases the excess risk of endometrial cancer but protection decreases with long term use of sequential regimens, and the risk is significantly increased after five years of use. [47],[48], [49]

The continuous progestogen regimens correct complex hyperplasia that arises during sequential therapy and keeps the endometrium suppressed in the longer term. [50]

HT and Ovarian cancer:

Although concerns have been raised about an association between hormone replacement therapy and ovarian cancer, studies have not shown a consistent increase in risk. For example, a recent study reported an increased risk of ovarian cancer in women taking postmenopausal oestrogen replacement therapy for more than 10 years (relative risk 1.8, 95% confidence interval 1.1 to 3.0) but no increase in risk of ovarian cancer among users of continuous combined hormone replacement therapy. [51]

1-3-5 Non Hormonal options:

- Exercise including walking programs, water exercise programs, keeping the core body temperature cool, paced respiration…
- Healthy diet and nutrition:

  The prevalence of hot flushes varies considerably around the world and is less in the Far East than in the west. Differences in diet and in particular the intake of phytoestrogens have been implicated and many studies have tried to establish whether dietary supplementation with phytoestrogens might be a suitable alternative to conventional hormone replacement therapy (HRT). Other lifestyle measures such as avoiding alcohol, caffeine and spicy foods may help. [52]

- behavioral strategies
- CAM: Different Complementary and Alternative Medicine (CAM) modalities and Menopause:

Concerns about the safety of Estrogen-based hormone replacement therapy after publication of the Women's Health Initiative study and Million Women Study has led to women turning to alternative therapies, believing that they are safer and 'more natural'.

In the most recent study by Kupferer and colleagues in 2009, the most common choices of complementary and alternative medicine were (a) multivitamins and calcium, (b) black cohosh, (c) soy supplements and food, (d) antidepressants, (e) meditation and relaxation, (f) evening primrose oil, (g) antihypertensives, and (h) homeopathy. [53]

Chinese Medicine and Acupuncture are the two widely used modalities of CAM between women who suffer from Menopause complications especially in China. This modality of CAM would be amplified in the next chapter.

Herbs like soy isoflavones, red clover isoflavones, black cohosh, also **vitamin E** are commonly used to treat VMS and may be considered in women with mild symptoms that are not controlled by lifestyle changes alone. [4]

Mind-body practices: In Menopause 2008, a study by Innes KE and colleagues reviews the effect of traditional mind-body practices such as **yoga**, **tai chi**, and **qigong** may offer safe and cost-effective strategies for reducing insulin resistance syndrome-related risk factors for cardiovascular disease in older populations, including postmenopausal women. Current evidence suggests that these practices may reduce insulin resistance and related physiological risk factors for cardiovascular disease; improve mood, well-being, and sleep; decrease sympathetic activation; and enhance cardiovagal function. However, additional rigorous studies are needed to confirm existing findings and to examine long-term effects on cardiovascular health. [54] A Systematic Review by Lee and colleagues in Menopause 2009 searched all types of clinical studies about the effect of **Yoga** for managing menopausal symptoms regardless of their design. It concluded that the evidence is insufficient to suggest that yoga is an effective intervention for menopause. Further research is required to investigate whether there are specific benefits of yoga for treating menopausal symptoms. [55]

The Study of Women's Health Across the Nation (SWAN) in 2007 released this information about usage of 21 types of complementary and alternative medicine (CAM) in midlife women: More than half of women used some type of CAM. Use of most types of CAM differed significantly by race/ethnicity, except the use of ginkgo biloba and glucosamine. Significantly more African Americans at most sites and Chinese women used ginseng. Use of most types of CAM did not differ significantly by menopausal status or vasomotor symptoms, except the use of soy supplements, which was significantly greater among women who reported vasomotor symptoms. Women reporting somatic symptoms were significantly more likely to use glucosamine. Women reporting psychological symptoms were significantly more likely to use ginkgo biloba and soy supplements. [56]

Evidence from randomized trials that alternative and complementary therapies improve menopausal symptoms or have the same benefits as conventional pharmacopoeia is poor. There are no recognized international criteria for the design of clinical trials of alternative therapies as there are for standard medicines and medical devices for endpoints of treatment and safety evaluations. [57] With the increased adoption of complementary and alternative medicine, it is important for health providers to be familiar with the various methods so they are comfortable discussing the benefits and risks with their patients to

assist them in making informed decisions. Also it is important to well-design research methods in the common methods of CAM.
Recently International organizations like WHO, also NCCAM are doing very well designed researches on CAM modalities.

Given patients' demands and utilization of CAM therapies, despite the lack of evidence, there is an increasing need to address how CAM therapies can be integrated into conventional medical systems. These suggestions should respond to patient's expectations and needs, but at the same time maintain accepted standards of medical and scientific principles of practice.

The effectiveness and long-term safety of alternatives to Estrogen need to be studied in rigorous clinical trials in diverse populations of women. This research is an attempt to fulfill this demand.

1-4 Menopauses from the view of Chinese Medicine:

In Chinese Medicine, Menopausal problems are fundamentally due to a decline of Kidney Essence which can take the form of Kidney Yin, Kidney -Yang or a combined Kidney Yin and Kidney –Yang deficiency. A combined deficiency of both Kidney Yin and Kidney –Yang in women over 40 is very common: indeed, it is probably more the rule than the exception.
Although a deficiency of the Kidney-Essence (in its Yin or Yang aspect) is always at the root of menopausal problems (with the exception of premature menopausal problems from Phlegm), other Full patterns often accompany it, notably Dampness, stagnation of Qi or stasis of Blood.
Chinese Medicine can help women to minimize their problems in the transition from a reproductive to a non-reproductive age. Herbal treatment is considered to be more effective than acupuncture reasoning that herbs are better at nourishing the essence. However acupuncture is an effective treatment for most of the menopausal symptoms that makes it to be considered as a safe treatment for lowering the burden of sufferings; despite the fact that it is not strong in nourishing kidney essence.
Generally speaking, if menopausal problems occur against a background of kidney-yin deficiency, the treatment will be more difficult; the redder and more peeled the tongue body, the more difficult the treatment.
Chinese medicine can help a woman in this transition period only in a slow and gradual way and its effects are not as rapid as those of HRT; but the potential impact of HRT on the risk of endometrial and breast cancer makes the alternative therapies such as Herbs and Acupuncture to be offered as options to the women in this stage.

1-4-1 Treatment of MRS by Chinese herbs according to syndrome differentiation

1-4-1-a Kidney Yin Deficiency and related syndromes

In women with menopausal complications, the deficiency of kidney yin should be considered, if they present these symptoms: Dizziness, Tinnitus, Malar flush, night

sweating, hot flushes, 5-palm heat, sore back, dry mouth, dry hair, dry skin, itching, and constipation.
Tongue would be Red without coating and the pulse is Floating-Empty, or Fine-Rapid, or very Deep-Weak on Rear positions and overflowing on both front positions.
The treatment principle is nourishing Kidney-yin, subduing yang, calming the mind and clearing Heart Empty Heat.
Suggested prescriptions are: Modified Zuo Gui Yin, Geng Nian Fang and Geng Nian An. Each of them contains a root part which nourishes the Kidney-yin

Sample formula	Herbs inside which nourish Kidney-yin	Point of emphasis	Suitable for
Zuo Gui Yin	Shu Di Huang, Shan Zhu yu, Gou Qi Zi, Shan Yao, Zhi gan cao	yin deficiency without much empty heat or heart empty heat	
Geng Nian Fang	Sheng Di Huang, Niu Zhen zi, Han Lian Cao	Nourishing Yin, absorbing fluids, calming the mind	Hot flushes with sweating and mental restlessness
Geng Nian An	Shu Di huang, Ze xie, Fu ling, Mu Dan Pi, Shan yao, Shan Zhu yu	Nourishes both kidney yin and kidney yang+ Blood and essence, but primarily kidney yin	Hot flush with cold feet

Some patent remedies would also be suggested; like "Qi Ju Di Huang Wan".

1-4-1-aa Kidney and Liver-yin deficiency with Liver-yang rising
The patient complains of irritability, dizziness, tinnitus, blurred vision, dry eye, dry skin, hot flushes, ache in joints, night-sweating, sore back, headaches.
The tongue may be red without coat; the pulse would be floating-empty, wiry on the left-middle position.
The treatment principle is nourishing kidney- and liver- yin, subdue Liver-yang, and calm the mind.
Suggested prescriptions: Kun bao tang, Qi ju di huang wan (a variation of Liu Wei Di Huang Wan), Qing xin ping gan tang

Sample formula	Herbs inside which nourish Liver- and Kidney-yin	Herbs inside which subdue Liver Yang or

		help that
Kun Bao Tang	Sheng Di Huang, Bai Shao, Niu zhen zi	Ju Hua, Huang qin, Suan zao ren, Long chi
Qi Ju Di Huang Wan	Shu di huang, shan zhu yu, shan yao, ze xie, mud an pi, fu ling	Ju Hua

Patent remedy: QI JU DI HUANG WAN

1-4-1-ab Disharmony between Kidney and Heart

This pattern consists of Kidney Yin deficiency with Heart Empty Heat.

The clinical manifestations might be as Hot flushes, **palpitations, insomnia**, night sweating, blurred vision, dizziness, tinnitus, anxiety, mental restlessness, backache, a malar flush, feeling of heat in the evening, dry mouth and throat, poor memory, dry stools.

Tongue: Red body without coating with a redder tip.

Pulse: Rapid-Fine, or Floating- Empty, or Weak Deep on both Rear positions and Overflowing on both Front positions.

Treatment principle: Nourish Kidney Yin, calm the mind, and clear Empty Heat

Suggested prescriptions: Tian Wang Bu Xin Dan, Liu Wei Di Huang Wan plus Huang Lian E Jiao Tang

Sample formula	Herbs inside which nourish Kidney- and Heart-yin	Herbs inside which calms the mind
Tian Wang Bu Xin Dan	Sheng di huang, Xuan shen, Mai men dong and Tian Men Dong	Wu wei zi, Dang gui, Bai zi Ren, Dan Shen, Suan Zao ren, Yuan zhi
Liu Wei Di Huang Wan plus Huang Lian E Jiao Tang	Liu Wei Di Huang Wan	Huang Lian E Jiao Tang (calms the mind by clearing Heart heat)

1-4-1-b Kidney Yang Deficiency

Clinical manifestations: Hot flushes but cold hands and feet, night-sweating in the early morning, pale face, depression, chilliness, backache, oedema of ankles.
Tongue: pale
Pulse: Fine, Deep
Treatment principle: Tonify and warm the kidneys, tonify yang, warm the centre, strengthen the spleen
Suggested prescription: You Gui Wan+Li Zhong wan. You Gui Wan tonifies and warms Kidney Yang. Li Zhong wan tonifies spleen yang which is necessary when tonifying kidney-yang.
Patent remedy: You Gui Wan

1-4-1-c Kidney Yin and Kidney Yang Deficiency
Clinical manifestations: Hot flushes but cold hands and feet, night-sweating, frequent pale urination, flushed around the neck when talking, slightly agitated, chilliness, dry throat, dizziness, tinnitus, backache.
Tongue: may be pale or red, depending on which deficiency predominants.
Pulse: Floating or Fine-Rapid if deficiency of yin predominates or Weak-Deep if deficiency of yang predominates.
Treatment principle: nourish the kidneys, nourish yin, gently tonify yang, calm the mind.
Suggested prescription: Er Xian tang+Er Zhi wan, Geng Nian Le, Geng Nian fang, Fu Geng Yin

1-4-1-d Excess patterns like "Accumulation of phlegm and stagnation of Qi", and "Blood stasis":
"Accumulation of phlegm and stagnation of Qi" is a pattern that appears in premature menopause in young women; in a few cases, menopause may arise not from a decline of the kidneys but from the obstruction of the lower burner.
Excess patterns should be treated by removing the excess element e.g. Phlegm, Qi stagnation, and Blood Stasis. [58]

1-4-2 Treatment of MRS by Acupuncture
Acupuncture, one of the oldest treatment modalities, is currently receiving wide publicity in the lay press and increased interest amongst postmenopausal women.

Definition and mechanism of action: Acupuncture originated in China 3500 years ago and works through stimulating certain points on the body by needle. The Chinese method is holistic, based on the concept that no single part can be understood except in relation to the whole body [59], and attention should be paid to maintain the body in harmonious balance within, and in relation to the external environment. Acupuncture is alleged to balance the harmony within the body. The stimulation of certain points on the surface of the body affects the function of certain organs, and those points follow a predictable and stable pattern. The acupuncture points are positioned along meridians, where a meridian is defined as `the line that can be drawn linking the points associated with any particular organ; meridians are channels for Qi. Qi flows through the body from meridian to meridian. Disease and pain occur when there is a blockage in the flow of the Qi. There are 365 acupuncture points, which lie along 20 meridians. Twelve of these meridians are primary, and correspond to specific organs, organ systems or functions; eight are secondary. To the Chinese, an organ comprises the organic structure and its entire functional system. It has been suggested that acupuncture might modulate the central nervous system and release of neurotransmitters. [60] Furthermore, changes in brain functional magnetic resonance imaging (MRI) signals have been observed during acupuncture. [61] a study reviewed the mechanisms of Acupuncture described that endomorphin-1, beta endorphin, encephalin, and serotonin levels increase in plasma and brain tissue through acupuncture application. It has been observed that the increases of endomorphin-1, beta endorphin, enkephalin, serotonin, and dopamine cause analgesia, sedation, and recovery in motor functions. They also have immunomodulator effects on the immune system and lipolithic effects on metabolism. Because of these effects, acupuncture is used in the treatment of pain syndrome illnesses such as migraine, fibromyalgia, osteoarthritis, and trigeminal neuralgia; of gastrointestinal disorders such as disturbance at gastrointestinal motility and gastritis; of psychological illnesses such as depression, anxiety, and panic attack; and in rehabilitation from hemiplegia and obesity. [62]

Acupuncture in managing menopausal symptoms:

Acupuncture was suggested to reduce the frequency of hot flushes by triggering the release of hypothalamic Beta endorphin, which is also partially responsible for a sense of well-being as well as having a pain-relieving effect. [63], [64] It is unlikely that acupuncture has a placebo effect, since it was previously reported that administration of placebo did not have an effect on the release of beta endorphin [65], [66]. Further, acupuncture was found to release 5-HT, which could relieve symptoms such as abdominal pain and cramps, mood swings and sleeplessness [63], in addition to its speculated key role in pathophysiology of hot flushes, as previously mentioned.

Safety of acupuncture in comparison with HRT:

Insertion of acupuncture needles causes minimal or no pain and less tissue injury than phlebotomy or parenteral injection, since it uses needles that are thinner than insulin needles. Acupuncture is safe when it is performed by experienced and well-trained practitioners, employing sterile and single-use needles. However, some adverse side-effects have been reported. [67] A study in Germany of 97 733 patients receiving acupuncture reported only six cases of potentially serious adverse events [67], including exacerbation of depression, asthma attack, hypertensive crisis, vasovagal reaction and pneumothorax. The most common minor adverse events included needle pain and local bleeding, both occurring in less than 5% of patients. [68] The needle size used varied between 0.2 and 0.3 mm, and there was no particular needle type or style that was linked to higher rates of adverse events. [69] One of the most common serious complications was the transmission of hepatitis viruses or other infectious agents via inadequately sterilized needles [67]; therefore, the use of disposable needles is essential. On the other hand, The Collaborative Group on Hormonal Factors in Breast Cancer, in their re-analysis of world-wide observational data, estimated that taking HRT from the age of 50 for more than 5 years would increase the risk of breast cancer by two extra cases per 1000 women [70]. Further, HRT was associated with a two-fold increase in venous thromboembolism, with the highest risk occurring in the first year of use. [71],[72]

1-5 Why should we do this research?

Menopause Related Symptoms are commonly experienced by women and involve the women's mid-life quality of life. MRS imposes immense psychological and socioeconomic burden on women's life. Current conventional therapy is Hormone Therapy. Concerns about the safety of Estrogen-based hormone replacement therapy after publication of the Women's Health Initiative study and Million Women Study has led to demand for other options; however, the efficacy and adverse effects of non hormonal therapies are unclear.

Among alternative therapies, acupuncture and Chinese herbal medicine are vastly required by midlife women. There are lots of studies about the efficacy of acupuncture or herbs in the treatment of MRS but most of them have methodological problems like lacking the control group or insufficient sample size of unclear methods which make these studies insufficient to give a definite idea about their efficacy. Moreover there are few studies comparing herbal medicine, acupuncture and Hormone therapy. And there isn't any well designed controlled trial comparing the effect of Kun Bao Wan with acupuncture and hormone therapy. Therefore, the current study would add great data to the literature by covering these shortages.

Chapter Two

Review of the literature

2-1 Kun Bao Wan in the treatment of Menopause Related Symptoms

There was no study about using Kun Bao Wan in the English data base. In Chinese Data base there were 5 articles about using Kun Wan in the treatment of Menopause Related Symptoms.

Wang Lei, et al. 2008: Wang Lei and colleagues in 新中医: "New Journal of Traditional Chinese Medicine", compared the effect of Meishen granules as the main intervention with Kun Bao Wan as the control. 60 perimenopause women with deficiency of Liver and Kidney or Disharmony between Heart and Kidney were randomly assigned in two groups. The outcome was changes in symptoms, FSH, LH and E2. The total effective rate in treatment group was 93.3%, control group was **86.6%.** The difference was significant (P <0. 05). the symptom score for Hot flash, sweating, insomnia and dreaminess, dizziness and tinnitus and the total score were significantly lower than the control group, the difference was significant or very significant (P <0. 05; P <0.001). In both groups after the treatment there was an increase in serum level of E2, compared with before treatment. The difference was significant (P <0.001). FSH and LH declined in different degrees comparing with before treatment; the difference was significant or very significant (P <0. 05, P <0.001). They concluded that Meishen granule is effective in the treatment of Perimenopausal women. [73]*Although in this study, KBW was used as the control group, but we can use the effective rate of KBW from this study which is reported as 86.6%.*

geng jia wei, 2002: Another study published in "Zhong guo lin chuang yi sheng" 2002, compared the effect of 3 months treatment by "Geng An tang" with "Kun Bao Wan" -as the control group- in women with menopausal symptoms. The Total effective rate of GAT was 94.8% vs. **70.8%** in KBW group. The total effective rate includes the patients who cured (40 out of 96 in GAT vs. 10 out of 48 in KBW) and the patients whose symptoms significantly declined although not totally removed (37 out of 96 in GAT vs. 15 out of 48 in KBW); and the patients who felt some effects but not significant (14 out of 96 in GAT vs. 9 out of 48 in KBW). 5 patients from GAT group and 14 patients of KBW group reported no effects by the treatment. [74] *Again like the previous study, KBW was used as the control group in this study, but we can use the effective rate of KBW from this study which is reported as 70.8%.*

Yan Hua, 2006: Yan Hua used Kun Bao Wan in combination with three other drugs for three different Chinese Medicine syndromes of menopause. He used KBW+Liu Wei Di Huang Wan in patients with Kidney Yin Deficiency (n=15); KBW + Jin Gui Shen Qi in Kidney yang deficiency (n=12); and KBW + Xiao Yao Wan (n=9) for patients with syndrome of Liver qi stagnation. Patients received the treatment for 2 months, 2 timed every day. The related article published in 2006 by "Zhong guo ming jian liao fa" indicates that total effective rate was 86.1% including 19 patients with completely cure and 12 cases who found it effective. The cure rate distributed in syndromes as followed: in Kidney Yin deficiency group, 8 patients cured and in 5 patients it was relatively effective. In Kidney yang deficiency group, 6 patients cured and in 5 patients it was relatively effective. In group with stagnation of Liver qi, 5 patients cured and in 2 patients if was relatively effective. The total effective rate (including all of the 19 cured cases and the 12 patients who found the treatment effective in all of the syndromes totally) is reported as 86.1%. [75] *the effective rate of combination of KBW and Liu Wei Di Huang Wan in patients with Kidney Yin deficiency syndrome in this study could be calculated according this reports data as 86.7%.*

An Rui Xian. 2008: An Rui Xian in "Xin yi xue zazhi" reported one case who reacted allergy to Kun Bao wan in 2007. The patient developed Urticaria in Chest, Abdomen and Back areas immediately after the first dosage. [76]

Xu jian.2006: There are many herbs in Kun Bao Wan. Looking for a "Quality Standard for Kun Bao Wan" in Chinese Literature, an article from University of Traditional Chinese Medicine, in Journal of "Chang Chun" was founded which suggested "Hunag qin dai" for evaluation of quality standards of Kun Bao Wan. This index should be more than 2500 to assume the product as standard. [77]

2-2 Acupuncture in the treatment of Menopause Related Symptoms

In this part, we review the articles found in English data base about the effect of acupuncture in the treatment of menopause related symptoms including 3 systematic reviews and 22 clinical trials.

2-2-1 Systematic Reviews about acupuncture for MRS

Lee et al. 2009: The latest released systematic review published in *Menopause* 2009 by Lee and colleagues from Korea included 6 randomized clinical trials (RCTs) of acupuncture versus sham acupuncture. They have searched the literature using 17 databases from inception to October 10, 2008, without language restrictions. They included randomized clinical trials (RCTs) of acupuncture versus sham acupuncture. Their methodological quality was assessed using the modified Jadad score. In total, six RCTs could be included. Four RCTs compared the effects of acupuncture with penetrating sham acupuncture on non-acupuncture points. All of these trials failed to show specific effects on menopausal hot flush frequency, severity or index. One RCT found no effects of acupuncture on hot flush frequency and severity compared with penetrating sham acupuncture on acupuncture points that are not relevant for the treatment of hot flushes. The remaining RCT tested acupuncture against non-penetrating acupuncture on non-acupuncture points. Its results suggested favorable effects of acupuncture on menopausal hot flush severity. However, this study was too small to generate reliable findings. They concluded that Sham-controlled RCTs fail to show specific effects of acupuncture for control of menopausal hot flushes. More rigorous research seems warranted. [78]

Alfhaily and Ewies. 2007: Another systematic review by F Alfhaily and A A A Ewies in *Climacteric* 2007 reviewed available evidence including 17 RCT (Randomized Controlled Trial), US (Uncontrolled Study) and PS.(Pilot Study) as regards the effectiveness and safety of acupuncture in treating menopausal symptoms. It concluded that the majority of women treated with acupuncture have a reduction of more than 50% in their hot flushes and this effect continued as long as 6 months after treatment, in some studies, with-out any adverse events. Despite these encouraging results, they stated that definitive conclusions cannot be reached because the majority of these studies are of poor quality, of small size, or used an inadequate control method; therefore, **doubt remains about their reliability** and the reported results could be entirely due to a placebo effect. They recommended that therapies purported to alleviate vasomotor symptoms should be compared with a placebo and an established therapy, since placebo treatment caused more than 50% reduction in hot flushes in the clinical trials that evaluated the effect of oral HRT. [79]

Kronenberg and Fugh-Berman. 2002: A systematic review by Kronenberg and Fugh-Berman in *Ann Intern Med* 2002 reviewed randomized, controlled trials of CAM therapies for menopausal symptoms. They Searched MEDLINE for articles published from January 1966 through March 2002, Alternative and Complementary Database (AMED) of the British Library for articles published from January 1985 through December 2000, and the authors' own extensive files. 29 randomized, controlled clinical trials of CAM therapies for hot flashes and other menopausal symptoms were identified. In their data synthesis, they mentioned that Single clinical trials have found that dong quai, evening primrose oil, a Chinese herb mixture, vitamin E, and acupuncture do not affect hot flashes; two trials have shown that red clover has no benefit for treating hot flashes. Other results of their review are about other CAM therapies. [80]

2-2-2 Clinical Trials about acupuncture for MRS

2-2-2-a: Acupuncture in healthy women with natural menopause

Avis, et al. 2008: A randomized, controlled pilot study of acupuncture treatment for menopausal hot flashes published by *Menopause* 2008 investigated 57 women ages 44 to 55 with no menses in the past 3 months and at least four hot flashes per day. They were randomized to one of three treatment groups: usual care (n = 19), sham acupuncture (n = 18), or Traditional Chinese Medicine acupuncture (n = 19). Acupuncture treatments were scheduled twice weekly for 8 consecutive weeks. The sham acupuncture group received shallow needling in nontherapeutic sites. The Traditional Chinese Medicine acupuncture group received one of four treatments based on a Traditional Chinese Medicine diagnosis. Usual care participants were instructed to not initiate any new treatments for hot flashes during the study. The results of this study shows that there was a **significant decrease in mean frequency of hot flashes** between weeks 1 and 8 **across all groups** ($P = 0.01$), although the differences between the three study groups were not significant. However, the two acupuncture groups showed a significantly greater decrease than the usual care group ($P < 0.05$), but did not differ from each other. Results followed a similar pattern for the hot flash index score. There were no significant effects for changes in hot flash interference, sleep, mood, health-related quality of life, or psychological well-being. Their results suggest either that there is a strong placebo effect or that both traditional and sham acupuncture significantly reduce hot flash frequency. [81]

Xia et al, 2008: Xia and colleagues evaluated the effect of electroacupuncture (EA) of Sanyinjiao (SP 6) on perimenopausal syndrome. A total of 157 PMS patients were randomly divided into EA group (n=81) and medication group (n=76) . EA (2/100 Hz, 8-10 mA) was applied to bilateral Sanyinjiao (SP 6), 3 times a week and for 3 months (mon). Patients of medication group were treated by oral administration of nylestriol, 2 mg/time, twice a month for 3 months. For PMS patients, medroxyprogesterone (6 mg/d, for 10 days) was added from the third month on after the treatment. The therapeutic effect was evaluated by using "symptoms-signs score scale", and changes of serum estradiol (E2), follicle stimulating hormone (FSH) and luteotrophic hormone (LH) were detected by chemiluminescence immune assay. Kupperman index was determined before and after the treatment. RESULTS: In comparison with pre-treatment, Kupperman index of EA group decreased significantly ($P < 0.01$). After the treatment, contents of serum FSH and LH of EA group decreased significantly ($P < 0.01$), while serum E2 contents of EA and medication groups increased significantly ($P < 0.\ 01$). Serum LH and E2 levels of EA group were significantly lower than those of medication group ($P < 0.05$). No significant differences were found between two groups in Kupperman index, markedly-effective rates and total effective rates ($P > 0.05$). CONCLUSION: EA of Sanyinjiao (SP 6) is able to regulate serum E2, FSH and LH levels and effectively improve perimenopausal syndrome. [82]

Qin, et al. 2007: A study similar to the former mentioned study by Qin and colleagues has been published in *Zhen ci yan jiu* 2007. They included 175 PMS patients (157 cases with complete data) were randomized into EA group (n=81) and medication group (n=76) according to multi-center (3 hospitals) and single-blind control trial method. EA (2/100 Hz, 8-10 mA) was applied to bilateral Sanyinjiao (SP 6) for 30 min, 3 times every week, with one month being a therapeutic course, 3 courses altogether. Patients in medication group were ordered to take nilestriol (2 mg, twice/month for 3 months) and medrysone (2 mg, t. i. d. for 10 days from the 3rd month on). Serum estradiol (E2), follicle-stimulating hormone (FSH) and luteinizing hormone (LH) were detected with a chemiluminescence immo-analysis system. After EA treatment, serum FSH and LH contents decreased significantly and serum E2 increased considerably ($P < 0.001$) compared with its basic values. Comparison between two groups showed that FSH, LH and E2 levels in EA group were significantly lower than those of medication group ($P < 0.05$). They concluded that EA of Sanyinjiao (SP 6) has a good regulative effect on reproductive endocrine function in PMS patients. [83]

Jin, et al. 2007: Jin and colleagues included 40 cases of PMS and randomly divided them into a treatment group who were treated with acupuncture at the five-zangshu and the control group with oral administration of Premarin tablets. The therapeutic effects and changes of Kupperman scores, and serum estradiol (E2), follicle stimulating hormone (FSH), luteinizing hormone (LH) levels before and after treatment were observed. At the end, the total effective rate was 90. 0% in the treatment group which was better than 65.0% in the control group (P<0. 05). After treatment, serum E2 level significantly increased (P<0.01), with a significant difference between the two groups (P<0.05), and with a significant difference between the two groups in Kupperman symptom score index (MI) after treatment (P<0.05). They concluded that therapeutic effect of acupuncture at the five-zangshu is better than that of Premarin for treatment of perimenopausal syndrome. [84]

Vincent, et al. 2007: Vincent and colleagues conducted a prospective, randomized, single-blind, sham-controlled clinical trial in USA which was published in *Menopause* 2007. A total of 103 participants were randomized to medical or sham acupuncture. At week 6 the percentage of residual hot flashes was 60% in the medical acupuncture group and 62% in the sham acupuncture group. At week 12, the percentage of residual hot flashes was 73% in the medical acupuncture group and 55% in the sham acupuncture group. Participants reported no adverse effects related to the treatments. CONCLUSIONS: The results of this study suggest that the used medical acupuncture was not any more effective for reducing hot flashes than was the chosen sham acupuncture. [85]

Zaborowska, et al. 2007: In *Climacteric* 2007, two prospective, parallel, randomized Swedish studies, involving 102 postmenopausal women, assessed the effect of transdermal placebo versus estrogen treatment (study I), and oral estrogen versus acupuncture or applied relaxation (study II), using the Kupperman index. It was found that the number of hot flushes per 24 h decreased significantly after 4 and 12 weeks in all groups except the placebo group. However, this trial did not include a placebo acupuncture control group. [86]

Ma, et al. 2007: Ma and colleagues from Shanghai explored the effects of acupuncture on granulocyte apoptosis and expressions of apoptosis-associated genes in the ovary of perimenopausal rats. The rats were randomly divided into 3 groups, including an acupuncture group treated with acupuncture, a medication group with Gengnian'an, and a perimenopausal control group, with young rats used for a control group. Granulocyte apoptosis and expressions of Bcl-2 and Fas proteins in the ovary of the rat were detected. As a result, Granulocyte apoptosis increased significantly (P < 0.01), expression of Bl-2 proteins decreased significantly (P < 0.01) and expression of Fas proteins increased significantly (P < 0.01) in the ovary of perimenopausal rats as compared with the young rats; after acupuncture treatment, granulocyte apoptosis decreased significantly (P < 0.05), expression of Bel-2 proteins increased significantly (P < 0.05) and expression of Fas proteins decreased significantly (P < 0.01); after treatment of Gengnian'an, granulocyte apoptosis did not significantly change ($P > 0.05$), expression of Bcl-2 prteins increased significantly ($P < 0.05$) and expression of Fas proteins decreased significantly ($P < 0.01$). They concluded that Acupuncture can inhibit granulocyte apoptosis, up-regulate expression of Bcl-2 proteins and down-regulate expression of Fas proteins in the ovary of the perimenopausal rat. [87]

Huang, et al. 2006: In a randomized, controlled pilot study, active or placebo acupuncture (placebo needles that do not penetrate the skin at sham acupuncture points) was administered to investigate the effectiveness of acupuncture on postmenopausal nocturnal hot flushes and sleep in 29 postmenopausal women, experiencing at least seven moderate to severe hot flushes daily. Acupuncture significantly reduced the severity of nocturnal hot flushes compared with placebo. The frequency of the flushes was reduced in both groups, with no influence on sleep. [88]

Wyon, et al. 2004: Another controlled study published in *Climacteric* 2004 randomized 45 postmenopausal women with vasomotor symptoms into three treatment groups: electro-acupuncture (n =15), superficial needle insertion (n =13) and unopposed 2 mg 17β-estradiol orally (n = 15) for 12 weeks with 6 months' follow-up. The mean number of hot flushes per 24 h, the Kupperman index and the general climacteric symptoms score decreased ($p < 0.001$) during treatment and remained unchanged 6 months after treatment ($p < 0.001$) *in all groups*. However, the curative effect of the superficial needle insertion, an inactive treatment, indicated that the positive effect of acupuncture was not more than that of the placebo. Moreover, the lack of non-treated controls made it impossible to know the percentage of women who had spontaneous cure within the 9-month period of the study. [89]

Cohen, et al. 2003: Cohen and colleagues conducted a small study stimulating specific acupuncture points related to menopausal symptoms (n= 8), while the control group (n = 9) had treatment designated as a general tonic to benefit the flow of Ch'i. Both groups received 9 weeks of treatment, followed by three no-treatment weeks. The treatment group showed a significant reduction in the number of *hot flushes and episodes of sleeplessness* when compared with controls; however, *mood swings were significantly improved in both groups.* [90]

Dong, et al. 2001: Another small study to evaluate the effects of acupuncture on the quality of life of 11 women with menopausal symptoms showed that it significantly improved vasomotor and other symptoms during **5 weeks** of treatment, and this continued for 3 months after the treatment. Nevertheless, there was *no change in psychosocial or sexual symptoms*. [91]

Grille, et al. 1989: Grille and colleagues randomly selected 45 menopausal women from two hospital clinics and divided them into three groups: HRT (n = 15), acupuncture (n = 15) and no treatment (n = 5). Groups one and two had comparable increases in serum estradiol levels. Nonetheless, the effect of both acupuncture and HRT wore off after stopping the treatment, and it was necessary to continue the treatment to maintain benefit. [92]

Di Conchetto. 1989: Di Conchetto reported **2 years** of acupuncture treatment of **100** women with menopausal hot flushes, with another 2 years of follow-up. They were divided into three groups, treated with combined acupuncture and moxibustion, electro-acupuncture, or acupuncture alone. Twenty women had complete remission, and 65 had a reduction in their symptoms. [93] However, it was an uncontrolled study, there were no formal outcome measures, and it was not clear whether the reduction of symptoms was assessed by the patient or the doctor. [79]

Limarti and Ricciarelli. 1989: In another uncontrolled study, 25 women with menopausal symptoms were treated for 1 year with combined acupuncture and moxibustion. Ten women improved completely, and the remaining 15 had partial improvement and reduction in their intake of sedatives or antidepressants. [94] In this study, there were no formal outcome measures.

Sotte.1989: In a case notes review of 238 women complaining of **joint pain associated with menopause** and treated with acupuncture for 8 months, 51% reported complete relief, 26% reported noticeable reduction in their symptoms, 13% reported accepted reduction in their symptoms but with tendency for recurrence, and 10% reported some improvement. [95]

2-2-2-b: Acupuncture in women with breast cancer and menopausal symptoms

Frisk, et al. 2008: Frisk and colleagues in their study which was published in *Climacteric* 2008, evaluated the effects of electro-acupuncture (EA) and hormone therapy (HT) on vasomotor symptoms in women with a history of breast cancer. 45 women were randomized to EA (n = 27) for 12 weeks or HT (n = 18) for 24 months. The number of and distress caused by hot flushes were registered daily before, during and up to 24 months after start of treatment. In 19 women who completed 12 weeks of EA, the median number of hot flushes/24 h decreased from 9.6 (interquartile range (IQR) 6.6-9.9) at baseline to 4.3 (IQR 1.0-7.1) at 12 weeks of treatment ($p < 0.001$). At 12 months after start of treatment, 14 women with only the initial 12 weeks of EA had a median number of flushes/24 h of 4.9 (IQR 1.8-7.3), and at 24 months seven women with no other treatment than EA had 2.1 (IQR 1.6-2.8) flushes/24 h. Another five women had a decreased number of flushes after having additional EA. The 18 women with HT had a baseline median number of flushes/24 h of 6.6 (IQR 4.0-8.9), and 0.0 (IQR 0.0-1.6; $p = 0.001$) at 12 weeks. Authors concluded that electro-acupuncture is a possible treatment of vasomotor symptoms for women with breast cancer and should be further studied for this group of women. [96]

Nedstrand, et al. 2005: A randomized study evaluated the effect of electro-acupuncture (n =17) and applied relaxation (n =14) for 12 weeks on vasomotor symptoms in postmenopausal women being treated for breast cancer. It was found that the number of hot flushes per 24 h was significantly decreased and the mean Kupperman index score was significantly reduced in both groups and remained unchanged 6 months after the end of treatment. [97]

Filshie, et al. 2005: A retrospective audit [64] of the electronic records of 182 women with breast cancer, who had 6 weeks of acupuncture treatment and were then taught to perform self-acupuncture weekly for up to 6 years, showed that 62.6 % gained $\geq$ 50% reduction in hot flushes and 16.5 % gained <50% reduction. The duration of treatment varied from 1 month to over 6 years, with a mean duration of 9 months. This study lacks a control group.

Porzio, et al. 2002: Another pilot study enrolled 15 tamoxifen-treated women with menopausal symptoms who were evaluated with the Greene Menopause Indexer. *Acupuncture improved anxiety, depression, somatic and vasomotor symptoms, but not libido.* There were no side-effects reported by any of these women. [98]

Tukmachi. 2000: Tukmachi reported a series of 22 consecutive women with breast cancer, referred for treatment of hot flushes, and who were given a course of classical body acupuncture for 7 weeks. The frequency of hot flushes improved significantly ($p< 0.001$) by the end of treatment. All women claimed some benefit and 82% had effective relief. [99]

Cumins, et al. 2000: In a pilot study included 21 tamoxifen-treated women with breast cancer experiencing vasomotor symptoms, acupuncture significantly reduced the frequency and intensity of hot flushes but not night sweats in 19 of these women. [100]

Towlerton et al. 1999: In a small uncontrolled study, Towlerton and Filshie reported that acupuncture treatment reduced the severity and duration of hot flushes in eight out of 12 postmenopausal women receiving tamoxifen for breast cancer. [101]

2-3 CAM in the treatment of Menopause

2-3-1 Frequency of CAM usage for Menopause Related Symptoms

Andrikoula and Prelevic. 2009: In the most recent review in English data base, Andrikoula and Prelevic in their review about Menopausal hot flush in Climacteric 2009 stated that in view of the contraindications and side-effects of estrogens and progestogens in postmenopausal women; however, there is a need to consider treatments other than hormone replacement for the relief of hot flushes. [102]

Kupferer, et al. 2009: Another article published in 2009 by Kupferer and colleagues, they found that **nearly half** of the 563 menopausal women who had discontinued the use of hormone therapy, used complementary and alternative medicine. [53]

2009: One survey has suggested that around **40%** of women in the **UK** have used complementary and alternative treatments for their menopausal symptoms. [103]

SWAN. 2008: There are really interesting findings in the recently released SWAN results in Menopause 2008. SWAN (The Study of Women's Health Across the Nation) is a prospective cohort study on the women from five racial/ethnic groups at seven clinical sites nationwide. Gold and colleagues in the year 2007 in Study of Women's Health Across the Nation in USA on 2,118 women, founded that **more than half** of women used some type of CAM and the use of most types of CAM differed significantly by race/ethnicity. [56] According to related article in Menopause 2008 by Bair and colleagues, approximately 80% of all participants (a group of 3,302 women) had used some form of CAM at some time during the 6-year study period. White and Japanese women had the highest rates of use (60%), followed by Chinese (46%), African American (40%), and Hispanic (20%) women. Overall use of CAM therapy remained relatively stable over the study period. In general, CAM use did not seem to be strongly associated with change in menopause transition status. Use of CAM among white women did not change with transition status. Among Chinese and African American participants, an increase in CAM use was observed as women transitioned to perimenopause and a decrease in use of CAM with transition to postmenopause. Among Hispanic and Japanese women, a decrease in use of CAM in early perimenopause was observed, followed by an increase as women entered late perimenopause and a decrease as they progressed to postmenopause. Patterns of use for the five individual types of CAM (nutritional, physical, psychological, herbal, and folk) varied. White women had relatively stable use of all CAM therapies through the transition. Japanese women decreased use of nutritional and psychological remedies and increased use of physical remedies as they transitioned into late perimenopause. Among African American women, use of psychological remedies increased as they progressed through menopause. [104]

Keenan, et al. 2003: In 2003, Keenan and colleagues stated that **46 percent** of the symptomatic women aged 45 or older (n= 2,602), used complementary/alternative therapy either alone or in combination with conventional therapies in USA. [105]

2-3-2 Efficacy and validity of CAM research in Menopause Related Symptoms

Nelson, et al. 2006: A systematic review and meta-analysis on nonhormonal therapies for menopausal hot flashes published in 2006 by Nelson and colleagues concluded that most of the trials on no hormonal therapies have methodological deficiencies, their generalizability is limited, and adverse effects and cost may restrict use for many women. This study suggests that these therapies may be most useful for highly symptomatic women who cannot take estrogen; but they are not optimal choices for most women. [106]

Umland. 2008: This study by Umland in 2008 also gave similar judgment about the unclear role of herbal remedies in the treatment of VMS, as clinical trial efficacy data are inconsistent and inconclusive. Nevertheless, this study believes that soy isoflavones, red clover isoflavones, black cohosh, and vitamin E may be considered in women with mild symptoms that are not controlled by lifestyle changes alone or those who cannot or will not take HRT. These herbal remedies appear to be safe when used for short durations (d 6 months). The recommendation by this author is a little different and includes wider range of patients than the former mentioned study. [4]

Kronenberg and Fugh-Berman. 2002: In this systematic review, 29 randomized, controlled clinical trials of CAM therapies for hot flashes and other menopausal symptoms were identified; of these, 12 dealt with soy or soy extracts, 10 with herbs, and 7 with other CAM therapies. Authors found that Soy seems to have modest benefit for hot flashes, but studies are not conclusive. Isoflavone preparations seem to be less effective than soy foods. Black cohosh may be effective for menopausal symptoms, especially hot flashes, but the lack of adequate long-term safety data (mainly on estrogenic stimulation of the breast or endometrium) precludes recommending long-term use. Single clinical trials have found that dong quai, evening primrose oil, a Chinese herb mixture, vitamin E, and acupuncture do not affect hot flashes; two trials have shown that red clover has no benefit for treating hot flashes. They concluded that Black cohosh and foods that contain phytoestrogens show promise for the treatment of menopausal symptoms. Clinical trials do not support the use of other herbs or CAM therapies. Long-term safety data on individual isoflavones or isoflavone concentrates are not available. [80]

2-3-3 Herbal therapy as a CAM for MRS

2-3-3-a Herbal formulations:

van der Sluijs, et al. 2008: A very well designed randomized placebo-controlled trial published by Menopause 2008, evaluated the effectiveness of a formula containing Chinese herbs and Cimicifuga racemosa vs. Placebo in alleviating vasomotor symptoms and improving quality of life (n=93). van der Sluijs and colleagues from Australia found no statistically significant differences in mean hot flash scores (product of frequency and intensity), Greene Climacteric Scale scores, and Hot Flash Related Daily Interference Scale scores between the placebo and herbal treatment groups after 16 weeks of intervention. [107]

Haines, et al. 2008: A 6-month randomized, double-blind, placebo-controlled study of the effect of Dang Gui Buxue Tang vs. Placebo in Hong Kong Chinese women, was published in Climacteric. 2008. Haines and colleagues in this study found overall no significant difference between Dang Gui Buxue Tang and placebo in the treatment of vasomotor symptoms in Hong Kong Chinese women, but Dang Gui Buxue Tang was statistically superior to placebo only in the treatment of mild hot flushes. [108]

Green, et al. 2007: A prospective, randomized controlled trial in the year 2007 assessed the effectiveness of professional herbal practice in the treatment of menopausal symptoms at one urban UK as a pilot study. Participants were block randomized into a treatment group (n = 15) who received a course of individualized treatment from one of three herbal practitioners, and control group (n = 30) offered treatment after waiting 4 months. The treatment group demonstrated a statistically and clinically significant reduction in menopausal symptoms compared to the control group. It concluded that the treatment package from herbal practitioners improved menopausal symptoms, particularly hot flushes and low libido. This offers evidence to support herbal medicine as a treatment choice during the menopause. [109]

2-3-3-b Herbal monotherapy

- **Black Cohosh**

Palacio, et al. 2009: A systematic review of clinical trials about Black cohosh for the management of menopausal symptoms by Palacio and colleagues published in Drugs Aging. **2009** concluded that the benefits of black cohosh in the management of climacteric symptoms remain to be proven because between 16 studies eligible for this review, many of them had conflicting results. Methodological flaws included lack of uniformity of the drug preparation used, variable outcome measures and lack of a placebo group. Case studies suggest an additional unexplored area of adverse events that also needs to be addressed. [110]

Newton. 2006: Newton and colleagues in Ann Intern Med. 2006 published the same conclusion: Black cohosh used in isolation, or as part of a multibotanical regimen, shows little potential as an important therapy for relief of vasomotor symptoms. They enrolled a clinical trial composed of 5 groups: 1) Black cohosh; 2) multibotanical with black cohosh; 3) multibotanical plus dietary soy counseling; 4) conjugated equine estrogen with or without medroxyprogesterone acetate; 5) placebo. [111]

- **Phytoestrogens:**

Lethaby, et al. 2007: A systematic review by Lethaby and colleagues published in Cochrane Database Syst Rev. 2007 compared 30 trials on the application of Phytoestrogens like dietary soy, soy extracts, red clover extracts and other types of phytoestrogen. There was no significant difference overall in the frequency of hot flushes between Promensil (a red clover extract) and placebo. Some of the trials found that phytoestrogen treatments alleviated the frequency and severity of hot flushes and night sweats when compared to placebo but many of the trials were of low quality and were underpowered. There was a strong placebo effect in most trials. There was also no evidence that the treatments caused oestrogenic stimulation of the endometrium (an adverse effect) when used for up to two years. Authors concluded that there is no evidence of effectiveness in the alleviation of menopausal symptoms with the use of phytoestrogen treatments. [112]

Adaikan, et al. 2008: Red clover isoflavones in the menopausal rabbit model led to significant improvements in bone density, tissue integrity, and vaginal blood flow with minimal effect on uterine weight. The study was done in Singapore by Adaikan and colleagues and published in Fertil Steril. 2008. [113]

2-3-4 Other CAM modalities for MRS

- Yoga

Lee, et al. 2009: A Systematic Review by Lee and colleagues in Menopause 2009 searched all types of clinical studies about the effect of Yoga for managing menopausal symptoms regardless of their design. It concluded that the evidence is insufficient to suggest that yoga is an effective intervention for menopause. Further research is required to investigate whether there are specific benefits of yoga for treating menopausal symptoms. [55]

- Mind-body therapies

Innes, et al. 2008: In Menopause 2008, a study by Innes KE and colleagues reviews the effect of traditional mind-body practices such as yoga, tai chi, and qigong may offer safe and cost-effective strategies for reducing insulin resistance syndrome-related risk factors for cardiovascular disease in older populations, including postmenopausal women. Current evidence suggests that these practices may reduce insulin resistance and related physiological risk factors for cardiovascular disease; improve mood, well-being, and sleep; decrease sympathetic activation; and enhance cardiovagal function. However, additional rigorous studies are needed to confirm existing findings and to examine long-term effects on cardiovascular health. [54]

- Healthy diet and nutrition:

Sturdee, et al. 2008: The prevalence of hot flushes varies considerably around the world and is less in the Far East than in the west. Differences in diet and in particular the intake of phytoestrogens have been implicated and many studies have tried to establish whether dietary supplementation with phytoestrogens might be a suitable alternative to conventional hormone replacement therapy (HRT). Other lifestyle measures such as avoiding alcohol, caffeine and spicy foods may help. [52]

There are lots of suggestions under research for treating MRS which are out of this thesis domain; like exercise, walking programs, water exercise programs, keeping the core body temperature cool, paced respiration, behavioral strategies...

2-4 Summery of Literature Review

In our literature review we checked more than 50 articles.

Five articles have been presented for application of Kun Bao Wan and its efficacy and safety in the treatment of Menopause Related Symptoms. They promise benefits of KBW but these findings don't seem reliable being unclear and having methodological problems.

Twenty five articles have reviewed the application of acupuncture for MRS including Systematic Reviews and Original Researches. Most of clinical trials seem very optimistic but systematic reviews are still doubtful due to methodological problems of most of the clinical trials.

Eighteen articles are about the efficacy and different modalities of CAM for the treatment of MRS.

We didn't find any study comparing Kun Bao Wan with either HT or Acupuncture in both English and Chinese database; there were 7 researches compared Acupuncture with Hormone therapy.

Chapter Three

Methods and Materials

3-1 Objectives

3-1-1 General objective:

Determining the effect of Chinese herbal medicine and Acupuncture on Menopause related symptoms in comparison with Hormone Therapy and determining the prognostic factors

3-1-2 Specific objectives:

1) To determine the therapeutic effect of KBW, Acupuncture+KBW and HT according to the difference between *Kupperman Index/ FSH/ LH/ E2/ number of symptoms* before and after the treatment and compare the therapeutic effect of 3 groups

2) To determine the therapeutic effect of KBW, Acupuncture+KBW and HT according to the difference in Symptom Severity Score of flushing in patients who had flushing, before and after the treatment and compare the therapeutic effect of 3 groups

3) To determine the therapeutic effect of KBW/Acu+KBW/HT in Perimenopause and Post menopause patients and compare the treatment response to KBW/Acu+KBW/HT between Perimenopause and Post menopause patients

4) To Compare the therapeutic effect of KBW, Acupuncture+KBW and HT in perimenopause patients

5) To Compare the therapeutic effect of KBW, Acupuncture+KBW and HT in postmenopause patients

6) To determine whether or not there is any relationship between responses to the treatment and "time distance from the beginning of menses irregularity to the beginning of treatment" in KBW group, Acupuncture+KBW group, HT group and total. (Determining the "time distance from the beginning of menses irregularity to the beginning of treatment" as the prognostic factor)

7) To determine whether or not there is any relationship between responses to treatment and "time distance from date of menopause to the beginning of treatment" in postmenopause patients in KBW group, Acupuncture+KBW group, HT group and total. (Determining the "time distance from date of menopause to the beginning of treatment" as the prognostic factor)

8) To determine whether or not there is any relationship between responses to treatment and severity of *hot flash/ insomnia/ weakness/ headache/ palpitation/ mouth dryness/ 5 zone hot sensation/ constipation* at the beginning of treatment in KBW group, Acupuncture+KBW group, HT group and total and comparing KBW, Acupuncture and HT. (Determining *insomnia/ weakness/ headache/ palpitation/ mouth dryness/ 5 zone hot sensation/ constipation* as the prognostic factor)

9) To determine the distribution of *hot flash/ paresthesia/ nervousness/ Melancholia (depressed mood)/ vertigo/ weakness/ arthralgia/ headache/ palpitation/ formication/5 zone hot sensation/ tinnitus/ low back burning pain/heel pain/ dryness and pruritus of skin/ mouth dryness/ urine amount and color/constipation/ eye dryness/ vaginal dryness/ sensitivity to hotness or coldness* before treatment in treatment groups separately.

10) To determine the variation in *Flashing/ insomnia/ depressed mood/ nervousness/ number of symptoms* with age (Sample Size=97): Is there any relation between age and severity of *flushing/ insomnia/ depressed mood/ nervousness/ number of symptoms*?

11) To determine the variation in *Flashing/ insomnia/ depressed mood/ nervousness/ number of symptoms* with educational level (Sample Size=97): Is there any relation between educational level and severity of *flashing/ insomnia/ depressed mood/ nervousness/ number of symptoms*?

12) To determine the variation in *Flashing/ insomnia/ depressed mood/ nervousness/ number of symptoms* with marriage status (Sample Size=97): Is there any relation between the marriage status and severity of *Flushing/ insomnia/ depressed mood/ nervousness/ number of symptoms*?

13) To determine the variation in *Flashing/ insomnia/ depressed mood/ nervousness/ number of symptoms* with "Time interval from the beginning of menses irregularity to the beginning of treatment" (Sample Size=97): Is there any relation between "Time interval from the

beginning of menses irregularity to the beginning of treatment" and severity of *Flushing/ insomnia/ depressed mood/ nervousness/ number of symptoms*?

14) To determine the variation in *Flashing/ insomnia/ depressed mood/ nervousness/ number of symptoms* with patient's age in which the menses irregularity happened (Sample Size=97): Is there any relation between the age of menses irregularity and severity of *Flushing/ insomnia/ depressed mood/ nervousness/ number of symptoms*?

15) To determine whether or not there is a significant difference between perimenopause patients and postmenopause patients in presence and severity of *Flashing/ insomnia/ depressed mood/ nervousness/ number of symptoms/ arthralgia* (Sample Size=97): Is there any relation between menopause stage and severity of *Flushing/ insomnia/ depressed mood/ nervousness/ number of symptoms/ arthralgia*?

3-1-3) Hypothesis of research:

1) There is no difference between the effect of KBW, Acupuncture+KBW and HT on decreasing *Kupperman Index/ FSH/ LH / number of symptoms.*

2) There is no difference between the effect of KBW, Acupuncture+KBW and HT on decreasing Symptom Severity Score of flushing in patients who have flushing

3) There is no difference between the effect of KBW, Acupuncture+KBW and HT on increasing the level of E2.

4) There is no difference between the therapeutic effect of *KBW/ Acu+KBW/ HT* in Perimenopause and Post menopause patients.

5) There is no difference between the therapeutic effect of KBW, Acupuncture+KBW and HT in perimenopause patients.

6) There is no difference between the therapeutic effect of KBW, Acupuncture+KBW and HT in postmenopause patients

7) There is no relationship between responses to the treatment and "time distance from the beginning of menses irregularity to the beginning of treatment" in KBW group, Acupuncture+KBW group, HT group and total.

8) There is no relationship between responses to the treatment and "**Time distance from date of menopause to the beginning of treatment**".

9) There is no relationship between responses to the treatment and **Insomnia/ Weakness/ Headache/ Palpitation/ Mouth Dryness/ 5 zone hot sensations/ Constipation .**

10) There is no relationship between the severity of *flashing/ insomnia/ depressed mood/ nervousness/ number of symptoms* and **age**.

11) There is no relationship between the severity of *flashing/ insomnia/ depressed mood/ nervousness/ number of symptoms* and **Educational level.**

12) There is no relationship between the severity of *flashing/ insomnia/ depressed mood/ nervousness/ number of symptoms* and **Marriage status**.

13) There is no relationship between the severity of *flashing/ insomnia/ depressed mood/ nervousness/ number of symptoms* and **"Time interval from the beginning of menses irregularity to the beginning of treatment"**.

14) There isn't any relation between menopause stage (perimenopause or postmenopause) and severity of *Flushing/ insomnia/ depressed mood/ nervousness/ number of symptoms / arthralgia.*

3-1-4) Questions of research:

1- What is the distribution of *age/ marital status/ educational level/menopause stage/ menopause reason* before treatment in all the patients and in treatment groups separately?

2- What is the distribution of *hot flash/ paresthesia/ nervousness/ Melancholia (depressed mood)/ vertigo/ weakness/ arthralgia/ headache/ palpitation/ formication/5 zone hot sensation/ tinnitus/ low back burning pain/heel pain/ dryness and pruritus of skin/ mouth dryness/ urine amount and color/constipation/ eye dryness/ vaginal dryness/ sensitivity to hotness or coldness* before treatment in all the patients (n=97) and in treatment groups separately?

3- What is the distribution of all of the symptoms in perimenopause patients and post menopause patients?

4- What is the average Age in the beginning of menses irregularity in all of the patients (Sample Size=97)?

5- What is the average Age of menopause in Postmenopause patients?

6- Which symptom is the most common symptom in all of the patients? (symptoms in order)

7- Which symptom is the most common symptom in perimenopause patients? (symptoms in order)

8- Which symptom is the most common symptom in postmenopause patients? (symptoms in order)

9- What is the average number of symptoms?

10- What is the average symptom severity score of *hot flush/ paresthesia/ nervousness/ Melancholia (depressed mood)/ vertigo/ weakness/ arthralgia/ headache/ palpitation/ formication* in all of the patients, in perimenopausal patients and in postmenopausal patients?

11- Which symptom has the highest symptom severity score in *all of the patients/ Perimenopause patients/ Postmenopause patients*

3-2 Study design:

3-2-1: Title:

Menopause Related Symptoms: Traditional Medicine (Acupuncture and Herbal Medicine) vs. Hormone therapy

3-2-2: Category of research:

This research is an applied research.

3-2-3: Type of study:

This research is a **clinical trial** which compares the therapeutic effects of KBW, ACU+KBW and HT in the treatment of menopause related symptoms.
Besides the clinical trial, the variation in menopausal symptoms with age, education, marriage, time distance from the beginning of menstrual irregularity have been assessed in all of the patients including the patients who didn't continue with the study project (n=97). Also the menopausal symptoms in perimenopausal and post menopausal women have been compared in the mentioned sample size (n=97). In fact, the latter mentioned two parts could be considered as **case- series** studies.

3-2-4: Method: This Clinical trial (Interventional) compares the efficacy of Chinese herbal Medicine (Kun Bao Wan) and acupuncture in comparison with Hormone Therapy. The case groups including KBW (n=22) and ACU+KBW (n=20). They were selected by simple non-probability sampling method among patients referred to Gynecology Out patient clinic of Dongzhimen Hospital for the treatment of MRS; if they meet the Inclusion criteria and excluded if they have any of the exclusion criteria. The inclusion and exclusion criteria are listed in the part A of this section. The Chinese Medicine Syndrome Differentiation was established by one Chinese Medicine Doctor in order to make an equivalent diagnosis. Patients in KBW group received this drug for 8 weeks. Patients in ACU+KBW group received KBW for 8 weeks plus 10 sessions of acupuncture free of charge in acupuncture clinic number 6 of Dongzhimen Hospital. The method of acupuncture was maintaining needles in 11 acupoints for 20 minutes each time without any manipulation, moxibustion or cupping. Acupoints are described in part of materials. The control group which was treated with Hormone Therapy included 15 patients. They received Conjugated Estrogen 0.625mg + Progesterone. The protocol is more described in part of materials.

3-2-4-a) Study design: Treatment, Randomized, statistician blind, efficacy study

3-2-4-b) Inclusion-Exclusion criteria

Inclusion Criteria:

1) Women 40+ years old
2) Being diagnosed as Peri or post menopausal syndrome by Western Medicine diagnosis according to this definition*:

   2-1: Subject must have rise in FSH (more than 10) or menses irregularity, also surgical post menopause is included

   2-2: must have at least 3 of symptoms mentioned in Kupperman Index

3) Being diagnosed as Kidney and Liver yin deficiency with Liver yang hyperactivity pattern according to Chinese.
4) Current users prescribed medications that influence hot flush rate (e. g. HRT, SSRI' s) were included after a washout period. The washout-periods was 8 weeks for SSRI' s and systemic HRT and 4 weeks for local Estradiol preparations.

Exclusion Criteria:

1) Systemic Hormone therapy in past 2 months
2) Using any other systemic drug or herb which may affect our treatment
3) History or evidence of significant cardiac, renal, metabolic, endocrine or hepatic disease or breast cancer.
4) Subject has a disorder or history of a condition (e.g., mal-absorption, gastrointestinal surgery) that may interfere with drug absorption, distribution, metabolism, or excretion.
5) History of Breast cancer or unknown breast lump, endometrial cancer, Thromboembolic diseases, uninvestigated vaginal bleeding and untreated Hypertension for HRT group
6) Currently breastfeeding

3-2-4-c) Enrollment: 57 patients in three groups (KBW: 22, ACU+KBW: 20, HT: 15) We calculated the sample size of clinical trial study according the previous studies.

3-2-5: Study duration: 2008 June 1- 2009 July

3-2-6: Location of research:

- clinic number 5, outpatient clinic of Gynecology, Dong zhi men hospital
- clinic number 6, Acupuncture outpatient clinic, Dong zhi men hospital
- Clinic of Dr. Wang Chao Hua, Outpatient clinic of Gynecology, Beijing University's People Hospital.

3-3 Outcome and variables assessment scales:

Primary outcome measures: Kupperman Index [Time frame: 8 weeks]
Secondary Outcome Measures:

- level of Hormones FSH, LH and E2
- number of symptoms
- Symptom severity Score of flushing

3-3-1: Modified Kupperman Index: It is the most important outcome in our research.

Kupperman index is a numerical conversion index and covers 11 menopausal symptoms: hot flashes (vasomotor), paresthesia, insomnia, nervousness, melancholia, vertigo, weakness, arthralgia or myalgia, headache, palpitations, and formication. Each symptom on the Kupperman index was rated on a scale from 0 to 3 for no, slight, moderate, and severe complaints. To calculate the Kupperman index, the symptoms were weighted as follows: hot flashes (×4), paresthesias (×2), insomnia (×2), nervousness (×2), and all other symptoms (×1). The highest potential score is thus 51. The score of hot flashes was based on the number of complaints per day: none (0), slight (<3), moderate (3-9), and severe (more than 10). KI sheet is attached to the appendix section.

3-3-2: Chinese Medicine diagnosis sheet:
It is designed to contain the symptoms that Chinese Medicine attributes to Menopause patients who have the syndrome of Kidney Yin deficiency. It is a diagnostic questionnaire including questions about the menses irregularity or stop, symptoms of menopause, symptoms of Kidney yin deficiency (like 5 zone hot sensation, low back burning pain, tinnitus, dryness of mouth and skin, little amount and yellow color of urine, dry stool, sensitivity to hotness,...), tongue and pulse of kidney yin deficiency which was checked by one Chinese Medicine Doctor for all of the patients. Chinese Medicine diagnosis sheet is attached to the appendix section.

3-3-3: Level of Hormones; FSH, LH, E2
The hormonal level of all of the patients in 3 groups was measured in Biochemistry laboratory of Dongzhimen Hospital before and after the treatment.

The algorithm of method is attached to the appendix section.

3-4 Ethical issues:

The written Consent was fully understood and signed by all of the patients before entering the study. All the information of patients has been preserved in the secret manner.

3-5 Data Analysis method

All of the research data were entered to SPSS 16 software in two separate files by researcher: 1- data of clinical trial study (n=57) 2- data of descriptive part on the larger sample size (n=97). The blind **statistician in Iran** analyzed the data. Kolmogorov-smirnov test demonstrated that Kupperman Index before and after the treatment; and KI differences were normal in all 3 groups. Therefore, T test and Variance Analysis are valid.

Data was analyzed with ANOVA, paired and independent sample t-test and chi-square test. Level of significance was 0.05.

3-6 Materials

3-6-1: Kun Bao Wan

- **Ingredients of Kun Bao Wan with their related traditional applications**

1. Ligustrum lucidum (nu zhen zi) 女贞子: tonifies Kidney and Liver Yin, clears heat and brightens the eyes
2. Paeonia veitchii (chi shao) 赤芍: clears Liver heat
3. Rubus chingii (fu pen zi) 覆盆子: it is astringent and benefits Kidney
4. Angelica polymorpha (dang gui) 当归: tonifies and moves Blood
5. Cuscuta europaea (tu si zi) 菟丝子: tonifies Liver and Kidney Yin also Spleen and Kidney Yang.
6. Spatholobus suberectus (ji xue teng) 鸡血藤: tonifies and moves blood.
7. Lycium barbarum (gou qi zi) 枸杞子: tonifies Blood also Liver and Kidney Yin
8. Zizyphus jujube (suan zao ren) 酸枣仁: calms mind by nourishing Heart Yin and Liver Blood
9. Rehmannia glutinosa (di huang) 地黄: cools Blood and nourishes Yin.
10. Scutellaria baicalensis (huang qin) 黄芩: clears Shao yang heat.
11. Chrysanthemum sinense (ju hua) 菊花: clears liver heat and pacifies Liver Yang.
12. Lyceum Chinese (di gu pi) 地骨皮: cools the blood
13. Eclipta prostrate (mo han lian) 墨旱莲 nourishes Liver and Kidney Yin, cools Blood.
14. Adenophora tetraphylla (nan sha shen) 南沙参: nourishes Yin, clears heat and moistens.
15. Morus alba (sang ye) 桑叶: clears liver heat and calms liver Yang.
16. Hordeum vulgare (da mai) 大麦:
17. Cynanchum atratum (bai wei) 白薇: cools blood and detoxifies.s
18. Anemarrhena asphodeloides (zhi mu) 知母: clears heat and nourishes yin.
19. Polygonum multiflorum (he shou wu) 何首乌: tonifies blood.
20. Dendrobium nobile (shi hu)石斛: nourishes yin and clears heat.
21. Paeonia lactiflora (bai shao) 白芍: nourishes blood and yin and calms Liver Yang.

- **Manufacturer:**Beijing Tong Ren Tang 北京同仁堂
- **Package:**500 Pills/ bottle x 12 bottles/ package x 10 packages/ box

(500 丸/瓶 12 瓶/包 10 包/箱)

- **Dosage:** 5 grams each time; twice daily with warm water

(5g/次 2 次/日 温水服用)

3-6-2: Acupuncture

Acupuncture was performed by one acupuncturist in number 6, Acupuncture clinic, Dongzhimen Hospital in order to make an equivalent method for all of the patients. Needles were retained for 20 minutes without any additional manipulation, moxibustion or cupping. Acupoints were similar for all of the patients including: Shen Shu [UB23], Xin Shu [UB15], Tai Xi [KD3], San Yin Jiao [SP6], Tai Chong [LV3], Lie Que [LU7], Zhao Hai [KD6], Guan Yuan [CV4], Yin Xi [HT6], Fu Liu [KD7], He Gu [LI4].

In Traditional Chinese Medicine there are these explanations for the functions of selected points: [LU7] and [KD6] nourish kidney yin and strengthen the kidney. [LU7] is the confluent point of Lung and Ren Meridians. [KD6] is the confluent point of Kidney and Yinqiao Meridians. The combination of these two points works well in the problems of throat, chest and lung like dry throat. [KD3] and [SP6] strengthen the kidney. [HT6] and [KD7] stop night sweating. [CV4] nourishes the kidney and strengthens the uterus. [LI4] calms the mind and regulates ascending and descending of qi. [LV3] is the Yuan source point of Liver Meridian and calms the liver. [UB23], [UB15] and other back shu points have been presented as effective points in the treatment of menopausal symptoms by previous studies.[84]

This protocol was obtained from the book: Obstetrics and Gynecology in Chinese Medicine by Giovanni Maciocia, a worldwide famous acupuncturist and Chinese Medicine Doctor who is a professor of Nanjing University, as well as a world wide well known reference; and his books are the textbooks taught in universities who teach Chinese Medicine in English language outside of China.

3-6-3: HRT Protocols

CE+medroxyprogesterone acetate (MPA) in one of these two protocols:

A- From the day 5 of each cycle: CE 0.625mg/d for 28days + MPA 4mg/d in the last 12 days of the 28 days.

B- CE 0.625mg/day + MPA 2mg/d, unremitting. This regimen is for the patients who do not want bleeding.

Both of them were given for 2 months.

Chapter Four

Results

Results from data gathering will be showed by tables in this chapter in 5 parts. The first part will present descriptive data while parts 2, 3 and 4 will give the analysis. The fifth part belongs to the results of descriptive study.

4-1: Characteristics of patients

Table 4-1: Mean and Standard Deviation of Age in treatment groups

	N	Mean	Std. Deviation	Minimum	Maximum
KBW	22	49.36	4.07	43	59
ACU+KBW	20	49.65	2.97	42	54
HT	15	47.13	3.70	40	55
Total	57	48.87	3.71	40	59

ANOVA shows there was no significant difference between 3 treatment groups about participant's ages (P=0.09).

Table 4-2: Distribution of Marriage Status in treatment groups

All of the participants were married except for one case in KBW group.

Chi-Square test shows that there was no significant difference between 3 treatment groups about marriage status (P=0.46).

Table 4-3: Distribution of Level of Education in treatment groups

		KBW	ACU+KBW	HT	Total
High school diploma and less than that	Count	4	3	1	8
	%	18.2%	15%	6.7%	14%
College and more	Count	18	17	14	49
	%	81.8%	85%	93.3%	86%
Total	Count	22	20	15	57
	%	100%	100%	100%	100%

Chi-Square test shows that there was no significant difference between 3 treatment groups about level of education (P=0.60).

Level of Education

		Frequency	Percent	Valid Percent	Cumulative Percent
Valid	junior high school	8	14.0	14.0	14.0
	speciallized training high school	5	8.8	8.8	22.8
	high school	22	38.6	38.6	61.4
	college	9	15.8	15.8	77.2
	bachelor	11	19.3	19.3	96.5
	Master	1	1.8	1.8	98.2
	PhD and more	1	1.8	1.8	100.0
	Total	57	100.0	100.0	

Table 4-4: Distribution of "Stage of Menopause" in treatment groups

		KBW	ACU+KBW	HT	Total
Peri menopause	Count	16	13	11	40
	%	72.7%	65.0%	73.3%	70.2%
Post menopause	Count	6	7	4	17
	%	27.3%	35.0%	26.7%	29.8%
Total	Count	22	20	15	57
	%	100.0%	100.0%	100.0%	100.0%

Chi-Square test shows that there was no significant difference between 3 treatment groups about stage of menopause (P=0.82).

Table 4-5: Distribution of "the reason of menopause" in treatment groups

		KBW	ACU+KBW	HT	Total
Natural menopause	Count	21	18	14	53
	%	95.5%	90.0%	93.3%	93.0%
Surgical induced menopause	Count	1	2	1	4
	%	4.5%	10.0%	6.7%	7.0%
Total	Count	22	20	15	57
	%	100.0%	100.0%	100.0%	100.0%

Chi-Square test shows that there was no significant difference between 3 treatment groups about the reason of menopause (P=0.78).

Table 4-6: Distribution of Severity of Hot Flash before the treatment in treatment groups

		KBW	ACU+KBW	HT	Total
without (0 times/day)	Count	1	3	0	4
	%	4.5%	15.0%	.0%	7.0%
<3times/day	Count	4	5	8	17
	%	18.2%	25.0%	53.3%	29.8%
3-9 times/day	Count	14	5	4	23
	%	63.6%	25.0%	26.7%	40.4%
> 9 times/day	Count	3	7	3	13
	%	13.6%	35.0%	20.0%	22.8%
Total	Count	22	20	15	57
	%	100.0%	100.0%	100.0%	100.0%

Kruskal-wallis test showed that there was no significant difference between 3 treatment groups about severity of hot flash (P=0.67).

Table 4-7: Distribution of Severity of Paresthesia before the treatment in treatment groups

		KBW	ACU+KBW	HT	Total
without	Count	10	5	14	29
	%	45.5%	25.0%	93.3%	50.9%
sometimes	Count	7	5	1	13
	%	31.8%	25.0%	6.7%	22.8%
frequently has stabbing pain, numbness	Count	5	8	0	13
	%	22.7%	40.0%	.0%	22.8%
frequently moreover severe	Count	0	2	0	2
	%	.0%	10.0%	.0%	3.5%
Total	Count	22	20	15	57
	%	100.0%	100.0%	100.0%	100.0%

Kruskal-wallis test showed that there was significant difference between 3 treatment groups about severity of Paresthesia ($P<0.05$).

Table 4-8: Distribution of Severity of Insomnia before the treatment in treatment groups

		KBW	ACU+KBW	HT	Total
Without	Count	6	2	1	9
	%	27.3%	10.0%	6.7%	15.8%
Sometimes	Count	9	8	4	21
	%	40.9%	40.0%	26.7%	36.8%
Frequently	Count	5	8	6	19
	%	22.7%	40.0%	40.0%	33.3%
Frequently and Severe, needs Sedatives	Count	2	2	4	8
	%	9.1%	10.0%	26.7%	14.0%
Total	Count	22	20	15	57
	%	100.0%	100.0%	100.0%	100.0%

Kruskal-wallis test showed that there was no significant difference between 3 treatment groups about severity of Insomnia (P=0.06).

Table 4-9: Distribution of Severity of Nervousness before the treatment in treatment groups

		KBW	ACU+KBW	HT	Total
without	Count	5	2	1	8
	%	22.7%	10.0%	6.7%	14.0%
sometimes	Count	12	7	7	26
	%	54.5%	35.0%	46.7%	45.6%
frequently	Count	5	7	6	18
	%	22.7%	35.0%	40.0%	31.6%
frequently, I can't bear it	Count	0	4	1	5
	%	.0%	20.0%	6.7%	8.8%
Total	Count	22	20	15	57
	%	100.0%	100.0%	100.0%	100.0%

Kruskal-wallis test showed that there was significant difference between 3 treatment groups about severity of Nervousness ($P<0.05$).

Table 4-10: Distribution of Severity of Depressed mood before the treatment in treatment groups

		KBW	ACU+KBW	HT	Total
without	Count	12	6	2	20
	%	54.5%	30.0%	13.3%	35.1%
sometimes	Count	8	6	9	23
	%	36.4%	30.0%	60.0%	40.4%
frequently but tolerable	Count	2	5	3	10
	%	9.1%	25.0%	20.0%	17.5%
Loses the life confidence	Count	0	3	1	4
	%	.0%	15.0%	6.7%	7.0%
Total	Count	22	20	15	57
	%	100.0%	100.0%	100.0 %	100.0%

Kruskal-wallis test showed that there was significant difference between 3 treatment groups about the severity of depressed mood ($P<0.05$).

Table 4-11: Distribution of Severity of Vertigo before the treatment in treatment groups

		KBW	ACU+KBW	HT	Total
without	Count	7	4	7	18
	%	31.8%	20.0%	46.7%	31.6%
sometimes	Count	9	9	6	24

	%	40.9%	45.0%	40.0%	42.1%
frequently, does not affect life	Count	5	5	1	11
	%	22.7%	25.0%	6.7%	19.3%
affects life and work	Count	1	2	1	4
	%	4.5%	10.0%	6.7%	7.0%
Total	Count	22	20	15	57
	%	100.0%	100.0%	100.0%	100.0%

Kruskal-wallis test showed that there was no significant difference between 3 treatment groups about severity of vertigo (P=0.19).

Table 4-12: Distribution of severity of weakness before the treatment in treatment groups

		KBW	ACU+KBW	HT	Total
without	Count	2	2	5	9
	%	9.1%	10.0%	33.3%	15.8%
sometimes	Count	12	9	5	26
	%	54.5%	45.0%	33.3%	45.6%
Frequently	Count	7	7	4	18
	%	31.8%	35.0%	26.7%	31.6%
The daily life is restricted	Count	1	2	1	4
	%	4.5%	10.0%	6.7%	7.0%
Total	Count	22	20	15	57
	%	100.0%	100.0%	100.0%	100.0%

Kruskal-wallis test showed that there was no significant difference between 3 treatment groups about severity of weakness (P=0.40).

Table 4-13: Distribution of severity of arthralgia/myalgia before the treatment in treatment groups

		KBW	ACU+KBW	HT	Total
without	Count	4	2	6	12
	%	18.2%	10.0%	40.0%	21.1%
sometimes	Count	10	5	8	23
	%	45.5%	25.0%	53.3%	40.4%
Frequently, but does not affect the function	Count	6	10	1	17
	%	27.3%	50.0%	6.7%	29.8%
Function restricted	Count	2	3	0	5
	%	9.1%	15.0%	.0%	8.8%
Total	Count	22	20	15	57
	%	100.0%	100.0%	100.0%	100.0%

Kruskal-wallis test showed that there was significant difference between 3 treatment groups about severity of Arthralgia/myalgia ($P<0.05$).

Table 4-14: Distribution of severity of headache before the treatment in treatment groups

		KBW	ACU+KBW	HT	Total
without	Count	9	5	11	25
	%	40.9%	25.0%	73.3%	43.9%
sometimes	Count	10	4	4	18
	%	45.5%	20.0%	26.7%	31.6%
frequently, but tolerable	Count	2	6	0	8
	%	9.1%	30.0%	.0%	14.0%
needs analgesics	Count	1	5	0	6
	%	4.5%	25.0%	.0%	10.5%
Total	Count	22	20	15	57
	%	100.0%	100.0%	100.0%	100.0%

Kruskal-wallis test showed that there was significant difference between 3 treatment groups about severity of Headache ($P<0.05$).

Table 4-15: Distribution of severity of Palpitation before the treatment in treatment groups

		KBW	ACU+KBW	HT	Total
without	Count	7	3	6	16
	%	31.8%	15.0%	40.0%	28.1%
sometimes	Count	8	6	6	20
	%	36.4%	30.0%	40.0%	35.1%
frequently, doesn't affect the work	Count	6	9	2	17
	%	27.3%	45.0%	13.3%	29.8%
needs treatment	Count	1	2	1	4
	%	4.5%	10.0%	6.7%	7.0%
Total	Count	22	20	15	57
	%	100.0%	100.0%	100.0%	100.0%

Kruskal-wallis test showed that there was no significant difference between 3 treatment groups about severity of palpitation ($P=0.08$).

Table 4-16: Distribution of severity of Formication before the treatment in treatment groups

		KBW	ACU+KBW	HT	Total
without	Count	19	8	15	42
	%	86.4%	40.0%	100.0%	73.7%
sometimes	Count	1	7	0	8
	%	4.5%	35.0%	.0%	14.0%
frequently, but tolerable	Count	2	4	0	6
	%	9.1%	20.0%	.0%	10.5%

needs treatment	Count	0	1	0	1
	%	.0%	5.0%	.0%	1.8%
Total	Count	22	20	15	57
	%	100.0%	100.0%	100.0%	100.0%

Kruskal-wallis test showed that there was significant difference between 3 treatment groups about severity of formication (P<0.05).

Table 4-17: Distribution of severity of Low back burning pain before the treatment in treatment groups

		KBW	ACU+KBW	HT	Total
without	Count	4	4	5	13
	%	18.2%	20.0%	33.3%	22.8%
mild	Count	8	12	9	29
	%	36.4%	60.0%	60.0%	50.9%
moderate	Count	9	4	0	13
	%	40.9%	20.0%	.0%	22.8%
severe	Count	1	0	1	2
	%	4.5%	.0%	6.7%	3.5%
Total	Count	22	20	15	57
	%	100.0%	100.0%	100.0%	100.0%

Kruskal-wallis test showed that there was no significant difference between 3 treatment groups about severity of Low back burning pain (P=0.08).

Table 4-18: Distribution of severity of Mouth dryness before the treatment in treatment groups

		KBW	ACU+KBW	HT	Total
without	Count	3	5	6	14
	%	13.6%	25.0%	40.0%	24.6%
mild	Count	8	9	8	25
	%	36.4%	45.0%	53.3%	43.9%
moderate	Count	9	6	0	15
	%	40.9%	30.0%	.0%	26.3%
severe	Count	2	0	1	3
	%	9.1%	.0%	6.7%	5.3%
Total	Count	22	20	15	57
	%	100.0%	100.0%	100.0%	100.0%

Kruskal-wallis test showed that there was significant difference between 3 treatment groups about severity of mouth dryness (P<0.05).

		KBW	ACU+KBW	HT	Total
without	Count	14	9	12	35
	%	63.6%	45.0%	80.0%	61.4%

sometimes has constipation	Count	7	7	3	17
	%	31.8%	35.0%	20.0%	29.8%
always has constipation	Count	1	4	0	5
	%	4.5%	20.0%	.0%	8.8%
Total	Count	22	20	15	57
	%	100.0%	100.0%	100.0%	100.0%

Table 4-19: Distribution of severity of Constipation before the treatment in treatment groups

Kruskal-wallis test showed that there was no significant difference between 3 treatment groups about severity of constipation (P=0.06).

Table 4-20: Distribution of "5 zone hot sensation" before the treatment in treatment groups

		KBW	ACU+KBW	HT	Total
Yes	Count	9	13	7	29
	%	40.9%	65.0%	46.7%	50.9%
No	Count	13	7	8	28
	%	59.1%	35.0%	53.3%	49.1%
Total	Count	22	20	15	57
	%	100.0%	100.0%	100.0%	100.0%

Chi-square test showed that there was no significant difference between 3 treatment groups about having "5 zone hot sensation" (P>0.05).

Table 4-21: Distribution of Tinnitus before the treatment in treatment groups

		KBW	ACU+KBW	HT	Total
Yes	Count	8	11	0	19
	%	36.4%	55.0%	.0%	33.3%
No	Count	14	9	15	38
	%	63.6%	45.0%	100.0%	66.7%
Total	Count	22	20	15	57
	%	100.0%	100.0%	100.0%	100.0%

Table 4-22: Distribution of Heel Pain before the treatment in treatment groups

		KBW	ACU+KBW	HT	Total
Yes	Count	5	6	4	15
	%	22.7%	30.0%	26.7%	26.3%
No	Count	17	14	11	42
	%	77.3%	70.0%	73.3%	73.7%
Total	Count	22	20	15	57
	%	100.0%	100.0%	100.0%	100.0%

Table 4-23: Distribution of Skin Dryness before the treatment in treatment groups

		KBW	ACU+KBW	HT	Total
Yes	Count	12	14	7	33
	%	54.5%	70.0%	46.7%	57.9%
No	Count	10	6	8	24
	%	45.5%	30.0%	53.3%	42.1%
Total	Count	22	20	15	57
	%	100.0%	100.0%	100.0%	100.0%

Table 4-24: Distribution of patient's self evaluation of urine condition (amount and color) before the treatment in treatment groups

		KBW	ACU+KBW	HT	Total
little and yellow	Count	3	6	4	13
	%	13.6%	30.0%	26.7%	22.8%
much and white	Count	0	3	0	3
	%	.0%	15.0%	.0%	5.3%
normal amount and color	Count	12	5	11	28
	%	54.5%	25.0%	73.3%	49.1%
much amount but yellow	Count	2	1	0	3
	%	9.1%	5.0%	.0%	5.3%
normal amount but yellow		5	5	0	10
		22.7%	25.0%	.0%	17.5%
Total	Count	22	20	15	57
	%	100.0%	100.0%	100.0%	100.0%

Table 4-25: Distribution of Eyes Dryness before the treatment in treatment groups

		KBW	ACU+KBW	HT	Total
Yes	Count	15	13	9	37
	%	68.2%	65.0%	60.0%	64.9%
No	Count	7	7	6	20
	%	31.8%	35.0%	40.0%	35.1%
Total	Count	22	20	15	57
	%	100.0%	100.0%	100.0%	100.0%

Table 4-26: Distribution of patient's feeling of Vaginal Dryness before the treatment in treatment groups

		KBW	ACU+KBW	HT	Total
Yes	Count	9	9	10	28
	%	45.0%	52.9%	66.7%	53.8%
No	Count	9	5	5	19
	%	45.0%	29.4%	33.3%	36.5%
Unknown	Count	2	3	0	5
	%	10.0%	17.6%	.0%	9.6%

Total	Count	20	17	15	52
	%	100.0%	100.0%	100.0%	100.0%

Table 4-27: Distribution of Hot/Cold Sensitivity before the treatment in treatment groups

		KBW	ACU+KBW	HT	Total
Sensitive to hotness	Count	7	6	4	17
	%	36.8%	37.5%	26.7%	34.0%
Sensitive to coldness	Count	7	6	8	21
	%	36.8%	37.5%	53.3%	42.0%
Sensitive to both hotness and coldness	Count	4	4	2	10
	%	21.1%	25.0%	13.3%	20.0%
No sensitive	Count	1	0	1	2
	%	5.3%	.0%	6.7%	4.0%
Total	Count	19	16	15	50
	%	100.0%	100.0%	100.0%	100.0%

4-2: Response to the treatment

Table 4-28: Mean and Standard Deviation of "KI difference" in treatment groups

	N	Mean	Std. Deviation	Minimum	Maximum
KBW	22	-8.59	6.005	-22.00	5.00
ACU+KBW	20	-14.55	8.46	-31.00	1.00
MHT	15	-11.13	5.80	-23.00	-5.00
Total	57	-11.35	7.27	-31.00	5.00

"KI difference"= patients' Kupperman Index after the treatment - patients' Kupperman Index before the treatment

Chart 4-1 Mean of KI before and after the treatment

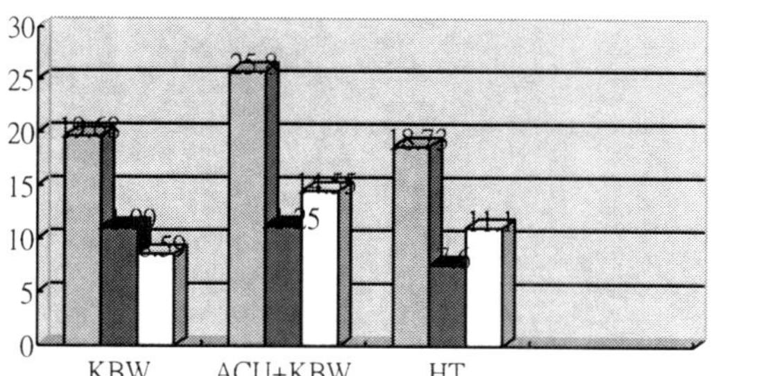

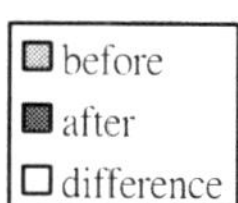

Table 4-29: T-test on the amount of Kupperman Index

	Kun Bao Wan	KBW+ACU	HT
Sig.	T=6.71 P<0.001	T=7.68 P<0.001	T=7.42 P<0.001

Paired T- Test in treatment groups demonstrates that each of them led to decrease in Kupperman Index of patients. (P<0.001 in every treatment group)

Table 4-30: Mean and Standard Deviation of the effect of every treatment on decreasing Kupperman Index

	Mean	SD
KUN BAO WAN	8.59	6.005
ACU+ KBW	14.55	8.463
HT	11.13	5.80
total	11.35	7.27
result	F=3.8 p-value=0.02	

According to one way ANOVA, the effect of three treatment groups on KI was different (P= 0.02). Tukey HSD test showed that this difference is between ACU+KBW group and KBW group. There isn't any significant difference neither between KBW and HT nor between ACU+KBW and HT.

Table 4-31: Mean and Standard Deviation of "FSH difference" in treatment groups

	N	Mean	Std. Deviation	Minimum	Maximum
KBW	16	-8.84	19.46	-58.10	19.40
ACU+KBW	19	-14.18	21.38	-51.80	34.50
MHT	15	-33.40	32.78	-78.84	31.54
Total	50	-18.24	26.39	-78.84	34.50

"FSH difference"= patients' level of FSH after the treatment - patients' level of FSH before the treatment

Chart 4-2 Mean of FSH before and after the treatment

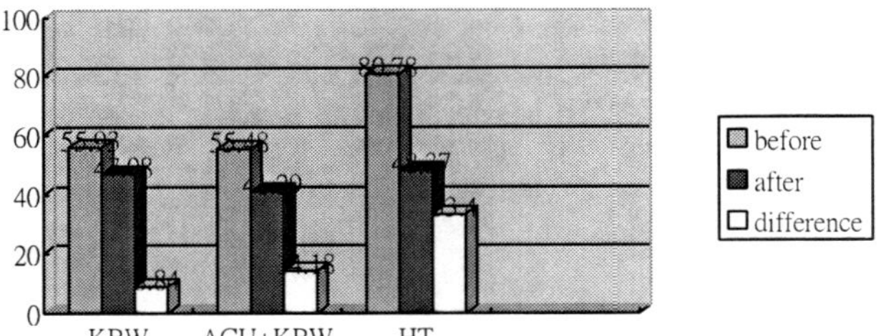

Table 4-32: T-test on the level of FSH before and after the treatment

	Kun Bao Wan	KBW+ACU	HT
Sig.	T=1.81 P>0.05 (0.08)	T=2.89 P<0.05 (0.01)	T= 3.94 P<0.05 (0.001)

Paired T- Test in treatment groups demonstrates that ACU+KBW and HT significantly decreased the level of FSH ($P<0.05$). KBW didn't make a significant decrease on the Level of FSH in patients. ($P>0.05$)

Table 4-33: Mean and Standard Deviation of the effect of every treatment on decreasing the level of FSH

	Mean	SD

KUN BAO WAN	8.84	19.46
ACU+ KBW	14.18	21.38
HT	33.40	32.78
total	18.24	26.39
result	F=4.198 p-value=0.021	

According to one way ANOVA, the effect of three treatment groups on the FSH level was different (P= 0.021). Tukey HSD test showed that this difference is between KBW group and HT group. There isn't any significant difference neither between ACU+KBW and HT nor between ACU+KBW and KBW.

Table 4-34: Mean and Standard Deviation of "E2 difference" in treatment groups

	N	Mean	Std. Deviation	Minimum	Maximum
KBW	16	26.90	96.61	-151.50	320.20
ACU+KBW	19	20.42	105.21	-215.10	274.20
MHT	15	27.83	50.47	-51.80	171.20
Total	50	24.72	87.54	-215.10	320.20

"E2 difference"= patients' level of E2 after the treatment - patients' level of E2 before the treatment

Chart 4-3 Mean of E2 before and after the treatment

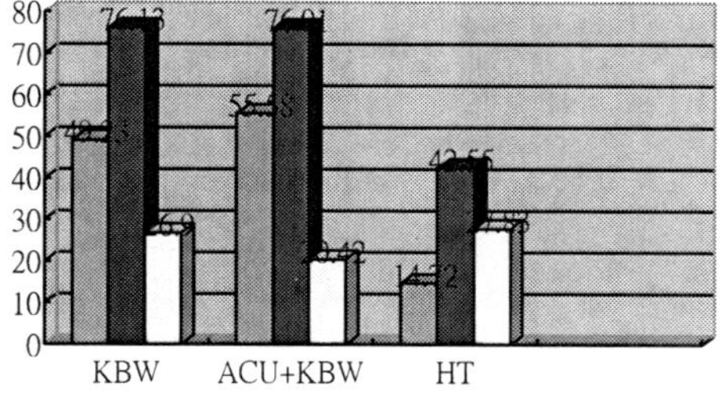

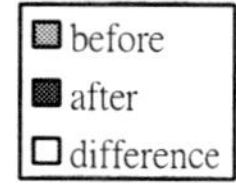

Table 4-35: T-test on the level of E2 before and after the treatment

	Kun Bao Wan	KBW+ACU	HT
Sig.	T= -1.11 P>0.05 (0.28)	T= -0.84 P>0.05 (0.40)	T= -2.13 P= 0.05

Paired T- Test in treatment groups demonstrates none of treatments significantly increased the level of E2 (P> = 0.05)

Table 4-36: Mean and Standard Deviation of the effect of every treatment on increasing the level of E2

	Mean	SD
KUN BAO WAN	26.9	96.61
ACU+ KBW	20.42	105.21
HT	27.83	50.47
total	24.72	87.54
result	F= 0.03 p-value= 0.96	

According to one way ANOVA, the effect of three treatment groups on the E2 level was not significantly different (P>0.05).

Table 4-37: Mean and Standard Deviation of "LH difference" in treatment groups

	N	Mean	Std. Deviation	Minimum	Maximum
KBW	16	-10.61	16.36	-53.60	14.90
ACU+KBW	19	-4.93	15.23	-33.20	45.34
MHT	10	-13.13	16.51	-48.70	4.69
Total	45	-8.77	15.93	-53.60	45.34

"E2 difference"= patients' level of LH after the treatment - patients' level of LH before the treatment

Chart 4-4 Mean of LH before and after the treatment

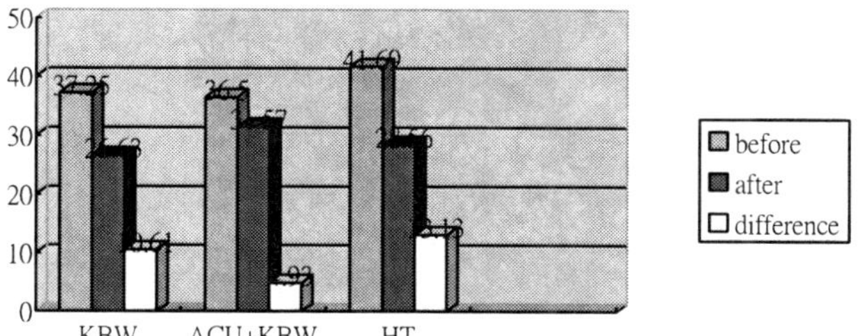

Table 4-38: T-test on the level of LH before and after the treatment

	Kun Bao Wan	KBW+ACU	HT
Sig.	T= 2.59 P< 0.05 (0.02)	T= 1.41 P>0.05 (0.17)	T= 2.51 P<0.05 (0.03)

Paired T- Test in treatment groups demonstrates that HT and KBW significantly decreased the level of LH (P<0.05). ACU+KBW didn't make a significant decrease on the Level of LH in patients. (P>0.05)

Table 4-39: Mean and Standard Deviation of the effect of every treatment on decreasing the level of LH

	Mean	SD
KUN BAO WAN	10.61	16.36
ACU+ KBW	4.93	15.23
HT	13.13	16.51
total	8.77	15.93
result	F=1.03 p-value=0.36	

According to one way ANOVA, the effect of three treatment groups on the LH level was not different (P= 0.36).

Table 4-40: Mean and Standard Deviation of "NS difference" in treatment groups

	N	Mean	Std. Deviation	Minimum	Maximum
KBW	22	-1.86	2.29	-8.00	1.00
ACU+KBW	20	-3.40	3.05	-8.00	3.00
MHT	15	-2.66	1.98	-6.00	.00
Total	57	-2.61	2.56	-8.00	3.00

"NS difference"= patients' Number of Symptoms after the treatment - patients' Number of Symptoms before the treatment

Chart 4-5 Mean of the Number of Symptoms before and after the treatment

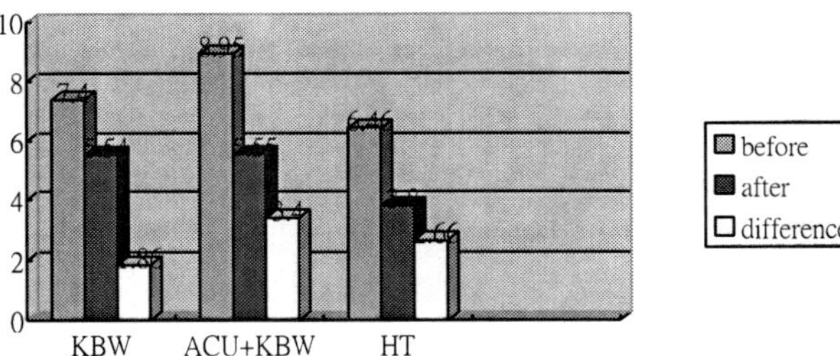

Table 4-41: T-test on the Number of symptoms before and after the treatment

	Kun Bao Wan	KBW+ACU	HT
Sig.	T= 3.80 P=0.001	T=4.98 P=0.00	T=5.19 P=0.00

Paired T- Test in treatment groups demonstrates that each of them led to decrease in patients' Number of symptoms. ($P<0.05$ in KBW group and $p<0.001$ in ACU+KBW and HT groups)

Table 4-42: Mean and Standard Deviation of the effect of every treatment on decreasing Number of symptoms

	Mean	SD

KUN BAO WAN ACU+ KBW HT	1.86 3.40 2.66	2.29 3.05 1.98
total	2.61	2.56
result	F=1.95 p-value= 0.15	

According to one way ANOVA, the effect of three treatment groups on Number of Symptoms was not significantly different (P>0.05).

Table 4-43: Difference in severity score of Hot flash after the treatment by every therapy

			KBW	KBW+ACU	HT	Total
HOT.DIFF	-3.00	Count	3	2	1	6
		%	13.6%	10.0%	6.7%	10.5%
	-2.00	Count	3	5	4	12
		%	13.6%	25.0%	26.7%	21.1%
	-1.00	Count	10	9	10	29
		%	45.5%	45.0%	66.7%	50.9%
	.00	Count	5	4	0	9
		%	22.7%	20.0%	.0%	15.8%
	3.00	Count	1	0	0	1
		%	4.5%	.0%	.0%	1.8%
Total		Count	22	20	15	57
		%	100.0%	100.0%	100.0%	100.0%

HOT DIFF= Severity of patient's hot flash after the treatment – severity of patient's hot flash after the treatment

Table 4-44:

	Patients group	N	Mean Rank
HOT.DIFF	Kun Bao Wan	22	31.59
	KBW + Acu	20	28.73
	HT	15	25.57
	Total	57	

According to Kruskal-Wallis Test, the therapy with less mean rank has had the best effect on decreasing the severity score of hot flash. Between the three therapies, HT has the lowest rank that means better decreased hot flash severity but the difference between treatments is not significant (P=0.500). Therefore the effect of KBW, ACU+KBW and HT on lowering the severity of hot flash has been similar according to this study. [114]

4-3 Response to the treatment in subgroups

Table 4-45: Mean and Standard Deviation of the effect of every treatment on decreasing KI in different menopause stages:

	Kun Bao Wan	KBW+ACU	HT	Sig.
	Mean ± SD	Mean ± SD	Mean ± SD	
perimenopause	9.68±5.81	13.30±9.74	9.09±4.06	0.26
postmenopause	5.66±5.98	16.85±5.24	16.75±6.70	0.008*
Sig.	T=1.43 P=0 .16	T=0.89 P=0.38	T=2.73 P=0.017*	

T-test shows that only in HT group there is a significant difference in decreasing KI between Perimenopause and post menopause patients ($p<0.05$); HT has been more effective in Post menopause patients. On the other round, Peri menopause patients respond to KBW better than Post menopause patients, however there isn't a significant difference between perimenopause and post menopause patients in response to KBW.

One way ANOVA shows that in Perimenopause patients there isn't any significant difference between three treatments' effect on KI ($P>0.05$); but in Post menopause patients there is a significant difference between three treatments ($P<0.05$). According to Tuckey test, this diference is between KBW and ACU+KBW (P=0.01); also KBW and HT (P=0.027). ACU+KBW is not significantly different from HT. The effect of ACU+KBW and also HT are significantly better than KBW in post menopause patients.

Table 4-46: Mean and Standard Deviation of the effect of every treatment on decreasing FSH in different menopause stages

	Kun Bao Wan	KBW+ACU	HT	Sig.
	Mean ± SD	Mean ± SD	Mean ± SD	
perimenopause	9.02 ± 14.41	16.04 ± 26.41	38.04 ± 32.14	0.02
postmenopause	8.30 ± 33.66	11.00 ± 8.60	20.65 ± 35.72	0.76
Sig.	T=0.06 P=0.95	T=0.48 P=0.63	T=0.90 P=0.38	

T-test shows that there isn't any significant difference between perimenopause and post menopause patients in response to any of treatments according to decreasing FSH ($P>0.05$).

One way ANOVA shows that in Perimenopause patients there is a significant difference between three treatments' effect on FSH ($P<0.05$); but in Post menopause patients there isn't any significant difference between three treatments ($P>0.05$). Tuckey test shows that the difference in perimenopause patients is between KBW and HT which HT is significantly better than KBW. The effect of ACU+KBW is not significantly different from HT and from KBW.

Table 4-47: Mean and Standard Deviation of the effect of every treatment on increasing E2 in different menopause stages

	Kun Bao Wan	KBW+ACU	HT	Sig.
	Mean ± SD	Mean ± SD	Mean ± SD	
perimenopause	32.45 ± 111.74	26.86 ± 132.32	35.88 ± 51.92	0.97
postmenopause	10.25 ± 19.94	9.38 ± 29.71	5.70 ± 44.86	0.97
Sig.	T= 0.38 P= 0.70	T= 0.35 P= 0.73	T= 1.02 P= 0.32	

T-test shows that there isn't any significant difference between perimenopause and post menopause patients in response to any of treatments according to increasing E2 ($P>0.05$). One way ANOVA shows that in Peri menopause patients there isn't any significant difference between three treatments' effects on E2 ($P>0.05$). The condition is similar in Postmenopause patients ($P>0.05$).

Table 4-48: Mean and Standard Deviation of the effect of every treatment on decreasing LH in different menopause stages

	Kun Bao Wan	KBW+ACU	HT	Sig.
	Mean ± SD	Mean ± SD	Mean ± SD	
perimenopause	11.63 ± 16.88	5.77 ± 18.41	15.35 ± 17.56	0.47
postmenopause	7.55 ± 16.65	3.50 ± 8.40	4.25 ± 9.82	0.85
Sig.	T= 0.42 P= 0.68	T= 0.30 P= 0.76	T= 0.83 P= 0.42	

T-test shows that there isn't any significant difference between perimenopause and post menopause patients in response to any of treatments according to decreasing LH ($P>0.05$). One way ANOVA shows that in Peri menopause patients there isn't any significant difference between three treatments' effects on LH ($P>0.05$). The condition is similar in Postmenopause patients ($P>0.05$).

4-4 Correlations

Table 4-49: Correlations between responses to the treatment and "time distance from menopause to the beginning of treatment" in post menopause patients

	Kun Bao Wan	ACU+KBW	HT	Total
	R (P-value)	R (P-value)	R (P-value)	R (P-value)
KI	0.03 (0.94)	0.01 (0.97)	-0.47 (0.52)	0.16(0.51)
FSH	0.58 (0.41)	0.79 (0.03)*	0.97 (0.02)*	0.40 (0.13)
E2	-0.87 (0.12)	0.03 (0.93)	-0.74 (0.25)	-0.07 (0.78)
LH	0.46 (0.53)	0.24 (0.59)	-0.39 (0.51)	0.22 (0.45)

About changes in symptoms (KI) by treatment, the correlation is negative ($p>0.005$).

About hormonal changes, in ACU+KBW group and HT group by considering FSH level as the therapeutic response, correlation is significant at the 0.05 level (2-tailed).

In all of the menopause patients in 3 groups, there isn't significant relation between responses to the treatment (according to KI, FSH, E2 and LH) and "time distance from menopause to the beginning of treatment" ($p>0.05$).

Table 4-50: Correlations between responses to the treatment and "time distance from beginning of menses irregularity to the initiation of treatment"

	Kun Bao Wan	ACU+KBW	HT	Total
	R (P-value)	R (P-value)	R (P-value)	R (P-value)
KI	0.06 (0.82)	0.12 (0.65)	-0.31 (0.49)	0.008 (0.96)
FSH	-0.17 (0.56)	0.17 (0.54)	-0.19 (0.68)	0.05 (0.75)
E2	-0.21 (0.48)	0.05 (0.85)	-0.27 (0.54)	-0.04 (0.79)
LH	-0.25 (0.40)	0.11 (0.67)	-0.91 (0.004)*	-0.009 (0.95)

In KBW group and ACU+KBW group by considering KI, FSH, LH, E2 as the therapeutic response, correlation is not significant ($p>0.05$).
In HT group by considering LH level as the therapeutic response, correlation is significant at the 0.05 level (2-tailed). This is a negative correlation.
In all of the patients in 3 treatment groups, by considering KI, FSH, LH, E2 as the therapeutic response, correlation is not significant ($p>0.05$ and r near 0).

Table 4-51: Correlations between response to the treatment and severity of Hot flash before the treatment

	Kun Bao Wan	ACU+KBW	HT	Total
	R (P-value)	R (P-value)	R (P-value)	R (P-value)
KI	-0.60 (0.003)*	-0.30 (0.19)	-0.59 (0.01)*	-0.46 (p<0.001)*
FSH	0.04 (0.88)	-0.05 (0.81)	0.006 (0.98)	0.03 (0.83)
E2	0.35 (0.17)	-0.20 (0.40)	-0.15 (0.58)	-0.06 (0.66)
LH	0.10 (0.70)	-0.22 (0.35)	0.44 (0.20)	0.06 (0.68)

In KBW group and HT group and in all of the patients by considering KI as the therapeutic response, correlation is significant at the 0.05 level (2-tailed) for KBW and HT; and at the level of 0.001 for the treatment totally. This is a negative correlation.

Table 4-52: Correlations between response to the treatment and severity of Insomnia

	Kun Bao Wan	ACU+KBW	HT	Total
	R (P-value)	R (P-value)	R (P-value)	R (P-value)
KI	-0.19 (0.39)	-0.45 (0.04)*	0.03 (0.90)	-0.27 (0.03)*
FSH	-0.36 (0.16)	-0.09 (0.69)	0.12 (0.66)	-0.28 (0.04)*
E2	-0.05 (0.84)	-0.20 (0.39)	0.05 (0.84)	-0.02 (0.85)
LH	-0.06 (0.81)	-0.35 (0.13)	0.64 (0.04)*	-0.06 (0.68)

In ACU+KBW group and totally, by considering KI as the therapeutic response, correlation is significant at the 0.05 level (2-tailed). This is a negative correlation.

Totally, by considering FSH as the therapeutic response, correlation is significant at the 0.05 level (2-tailed). This is a negative correlation.

In HT group, by considering LH as the therapeutic response, correlation is significant at the 0.05 level (2-tailed). This is a direct correlation.

Table 4-53: Correlations between response to the treatment and severity of Weakness

	Kun Bao Wan	ACU+KBW	HT	Total
	R (P-value)	R (P-value)	R (P-value)	R (P-value)
KI	-0.39 (0.06)	-0.29 (0.21)	-0.49 (0.06)	-0.38 (0.003)*
FSH	-0.16 (0.53)	0.24 (0.31)	0.14 (0.60)	0.15 (0.29)
E2	-0.13 (0.61)	-0.39 (0.09)	-0.009 (0.97)	-0.23 (0.10)
LH	-0.32 (0.22)	-0.31 (0.18)	0.20 (0.56)	-0.13 (0.38)

Totally, by considering KI as the therapeutic response, correlation is significant at the 0.05 level (2-tailed). This is a negative correlation.
About hormonal changes, correlation is not significant ($p>0.05$).

Table 4-54: Correlations between response to the treatment and severity of Palpitation

	Kun Bao Wan	ACU+KBW	HT	Total
	R (P-value)	R (P-value)	R (P-value)	R (P-value)
KI	-0.39 (0.06)	-0.70 (0.001)*	-0.35 (0.19)	-0.56 (<0.001)*
FSH	-0.05 (0.84)	0.02 (0.93)	0.47 (0.07)	0.20 (0.14)
E2	0.11 (0.66)	-0.13 (0.59)	-0.34 (0.20)	-0.17 (0.22)

LH	-0.16 (0.54)	-0.15 (0.54)	0.35 (0.31)	-0.01 (0.92)

Totally, by considering KI as the therapeutic response, correlation is significant at the 0.001 level (2-tailed). This is a negative correlation.
In ACU+KBW group, by considering KI as the therapeutic response, correlation is significant at the 0.05 level (2-tailed). This is a negative correlation.

About hormonal changes, correlation is not significant (p>0.05).

Table 4-55: Mean and Standard Deviation of KI in patients with or without 5 zone hot sensations in treatment groups

		N	Mean	Std. Deviation	Sig
KBW	YES	9	-11.77	5.49	T=-2.26
	No	13	-6.38	5.48	P =0.03*
ACU+KBW	YES	13	-16.15	9.39	T= -1.16
	No	7	-11.57	5.85	P= 0.25
HT	YES	7	-13.00	5.47	T= -1.18
	No	8	-9.50	5.92	P= 0.25
Total	YES	29	-14.03	7.54	T= -3.03
	No	28	-8.57	5.91	P= .004*

According to t-test, there is a significant difference between decreasing KI in patients who had "5 zone hot sensations" or didn't have this symptom in 3 treatment groups (p<0.05). In KBW group, patients who had 5ZHS respond better to the treatment and KI decreased in them significantly better than the patients without 5ZHS (p<0.05). In ACU+KBW group and in HT group the condition was the same but the difference was not significant (p>0.05).

Table 4-56: Correlations between response to the treatment and severity of Constipation

	Kun Bao Wan	ACU+KBW	HT	Total
	R (P-value)	R (P-value)	R (P-value)	R (P-value)
KI	0.05 (0.81)	-0.23 (0.32)	0.09 (0.73)	-0.11 (0.37)
FSH	0.00 (1.00)	0.33 (0.16)	0.11 (0.68)	0.19 (0.18)
E2	-0.16 (0.55)	-0.53 (0.01)*	0.07 (0.78)	-0.30 (0.03)*
LH	0.16 (0.55)	-0.53 (0.01)*	0.52 (0.12)	-0.008 (0.95)

About changes in symptoms (KI), correlation is not significant (p>0.05).

About hormonal changes, in ACU+KBW group and totally, by considering E2 as the therapeutic response, correlation is significant at the 0.05 level (2-tailed). This is a negative correlation. Also in ACU+KBW group, by considering LH as the therapeutic response, correlation is significant at the 0.05 level (2-tailed). This is a negative correlation.

4-5 Results of the descriptive study

The mean age in which menses irregularity has been started was 46.50 ± 4.42 (Min=33, Max= 57).
The mean age in which menopause has happened was 47.36 ± 4.30 (Min=37, Max= 54).
The mean number of symptoms in all of the patients was 7.61 ±2.38 (Min=3, Max= 11).
Totally the most common symptom in patients was Hot flash (92.8%). After that Insomnia (83.5%), weakness (82.5%) and Nervousness (81.4%) were more common. Other symptoms were in this in order: arthralgia (75.3%), palpitation (69.1%), vertigo (64.9%), depressed mood (62.9%), headache (60.8%), paresthesia (52.6%) and formication (29.8%).
In Perimenopause patients the most common symptoms were hot flash (91%), insomnia and weakness (79.1%) and nervousness (77.6%). Other symptoms were in this order in perimenopause patients: arthralgia (67.2%), depressed mood and palpitation (62.7%), vertigo (56.7%), headache (55.2%), paresthesia (46.3%) and formication (25.4%).
In Postmenopause patients the most common symptoms were hot flash (96.7%), insomnia and arthralgia (93.3%) and nervousness and weakness (90%). Other symptoms were in this order in postmenopause patients: palpitation and vertigo (83.3%), headache (73.3%), paresthesia (66.7%), depressed mood (63.3%) and formication (36.7%).

One-Sample Kolmogorov-Smirnov Test showed that age was normal so, Analysis of Variance Analysis is valid. Mean age of all of the patients was 48.90 ± 4.37.

According to one way ANOVA test, there was no relation between age and severity of hot flash (p=0.33), Insomnia (p=0.38), Nervousness (p=0.80) and depressed mood (p=0.42) but correlation between age and number of symptoms was significant at the 0.05 level (p=0.01, r =0.24).

Table 4-57: Distribution of educational level in patients with different severities of hot flash

		without (0 times/day)	<3times/day	3-9 times/day	> 9 times/day	Total
junior high school	Count	0	1	5	2	8
	%	0.0%	12.5%	62.5%	25.0%	100.0%
speciallized training high school	Count	0	4	4	3	11
	%	0.0%	36.4%	36.4%	27.3%	100.0%
high school	Count	3	8	8	12	31
	%	9.7%	25.8%	25.8%	38.7%	100.0%
college	Count	1	15	8	2	14
	%	7.1%	53.6%	57.1%	14.3%	100.0%
bachelor and higher	Count	1	15	7	5	28
	%	3.6%	53.6%	25.0%	17.9%	100.0%

Total	Count	5	31	32	24	92
	%	5.4%	33.7%	34.8%	26.1%	100.0%

To find out the relation between educational level and severity of hot flash, Kendall's tau-c test was done. It demonstrated that there is a significant negative relation between level of education and severity of hot flash (r = -0.165, sig=0.03).

The same test showed no relation between educational level and severity of paresthesia (r = -0.15, sig=0.05), Insomnia (r = -0.02, sig=0.78), Nervousness (r = -0.05, sig= 0.51) and depressed mood (r = 0.00, sig = 1.00).

Table 4-58: Mean and Standard Deviation of number of symptoms in different educational levels

	N	Mean	Standard Deviation	Minimum	Maximum
junior high school	8	7.62	2.32	4.00	10.00
speciallized training high school	11	8.00	2.48	4.00	11.00
high school	31	8.41	2.46	3.00	11.00
college	14	8.28	2.01	6.00	11.00
bachelor and higher	28	6.53	1.99	3.00	11.00
Total	92	7.70	2.34	3.00	11.00

ANOVA one way test established that there was significant relation between educational level and number of symptoms (F=2.949, p=0 .02). Tukey HSD test indicated that the difference in number of symptoms was only between "patients with high school diploma" and "patients with bachelor or higher degree".

One way ANOVA didn't find a relation between "Time interval from the beginning of menses irregularity to the beginning of treatment" and severity of Flushing (F=0.52, p=0.66), insomnia (F=1.13, p=0.34), depressed mood (F=0.56, p=0.63), nervousness (F=1.48, p=0.22). there was no correlation between "Time interval from the beginning of menses irregularity to the beginning of treatment" and number of symptoms (r=0.09, p=0.42).

One way ANOVA didn't find a relation between "patient's age in which the menses irregularity happened" and severity of hot flash (F=1.76, p=0.16), insomnia (F=0.93, p=0.42), depressed mood (F=0.45, p=0.71), nervousness (F=0.70, p=0.55). there was no correlation between "patient's age in which the menses irregularity happened" and number of symptoms (r=0.14, p=0.24).

In order to determine whether or not there is a significant difference between perimenopause patients and postmenopause patients in presence and severity of major symptoms, we compared the severity of hot flash, insomnia, depressed mood, nervousness, arthralgia in two groups of menopause stage (perimenopuase and post menopause) by Mann-Whitney test. We found a significant relation between relation between menopause stage and severity of arthralgia (p=0.003).

T test determined the correlation between stage of menopause and patients' number of symptoms (T= -3.22, p=0.002). It means that post menopause patients have significantly more symptoms than perimenopause patients.

Table 4-59: Mean and Standard Deviation of number of symptoms in peri and post menopause patients

		N	Mean	Std. Deviation
stage of menopause	perimenopause	67	7.1045	2.43792
	post menopause	30	8.7333	1.94641

Table 4-60: Mean and Standard Deviation of symptom severity score in peri and post menopause patients and totally (1)

	Patient's severity of hot flash	Patient's severity of paresthesia	Patient's severity of insomnia	Patient's severity of nervousness	Patient's severity of Depressed mood
Perimenopause	2.72±0.95	1.7±0.87	2.37±0.91	2.21±0.82	1.82±0.77
Postmenopause	2.83±0.83	2.17±1.02	2.5±0.86	2.47±0.93	2±1.01
Total	2.75±0.91	1.85±0.93	2.41±0.89	2.29±0.86	1.88±0.85
sig	P=0.58	P=0.02*	P=0.70	P=0.33	0.59

Table 4-61: Mean and Standard Deviation of symptom severity score (SSC) in peri and post menopause patients and totally (2)

	vertigo	weakness	arthralgia/myalgia	headache	palpitation	formication

Perimenopause	1.87±0.91	2.19±0.82	2.03±0.90	1.87±0.85	1.93±0.85	1.39±0.73
Postmenopause	2.17±0.74	2.53±0.86	2.6±0.77	2.30±1.08	2.47±0.97	1.5±0.73
Total	1.96±0.87	2.3±0.84	2.21±0.90	1.94±0.95	2.09±0.92	1.42±0.73
sig	P=0.05	P=0.08	P=0.003*	P=0.02*	P=0.01*	P=0.32

There was a significant difference in symptom severity score of paresthesia, arthralgia/myalgia, headache and palpitation between perimenopause and post menopause patients ($p<0.05$). These symptoms were more severe in post menopause patients than perimenopause patients.

Ranking by Mann Whitney test put the symptoms according to Mean Symptom Severity Score in this order in peri and post menopause patients:
Perimenopause: Insomnia, Depressed mood, Hot flash, Formication, Nervousness, Weakness, Vertigo, Paresthesia, Headache, Palpitation, Arthralgia/myalgia
Post menopause: Arthralgia, Palpitation, Headache, Paresthesia, Vertigo, Weakness, Nervousness, formication, Hot flash, Depressed mood, Insomnia

Chapter Five

Discussion

5-1 Analysis of the statistics and describing the results

We divided patients with MRS to three treatment groups: Kun Bao Wan, Acupuncture+Kun Bao Wan, and Hormone Therapy and evaluated their response to each treatment by means of changes in patients' Kupperman Index, FSH, LH, E2 and number of symptoms.

The statistical analysis would be discussed here in three parts: first of all, the therapeutic response in three treatment groups (KBW, ACU+KBW, and HT); then the therapeutic response in subgroups (peri menopause patients vs. post menopause patients) and finally the correlations found between treatment response and symptoms or conditions of the patients.

5-1-1 the therapeutic response in three treatment groups

5-1-1-1: According to decrease in KI:

- KBW is effective in the treatment of MRS ($P<0.001$).
- ACU + KBW is effective in the treatment of MRS ($P<0.001$).
- HT is effective in the treatment of MRS ($P<0.001$).

- The effect of three treatments were significantly different according to ANOVA test ($p<0.05$). This difference is between ACU+KBW group and KBW group according to Tukey HSD test. The effect of ACU + KBW is significantly better than KBW in decreasing KI ($P<0.05$).
- There isn't any significant difference between the effect of KBW and HT.
- There isn't any significant difference between the effect of ACU+KBW and HT.

5-1-1-2:According to decrease in the level of FSH:

- KBW didn't make a significant decrease in the Level of FSH in patients. ($P>0.05$)
- Both of ACU+KBW and HT significantly decreased the level of FSH ($P<0.05$).

- According to one way ANOVA, the effect of three treatment groups on the FSH level was different ($P= 0.021$). Tukey HSD test showed that this difference is between KBW group and HT group. HT was significantly better than KBW in decreasing FSH ($P<0.05$).
- There isn't any significant difference between the effect of HT and ACU + KBW in decreasing FSH
- There isn't any significant difference between the effect of KBW and ACU + KBW in decreasing FSH

5-1-1-3:According to increase in the level of E2:

- KBW, ACU + KBW and HT didn't make any significant increase in the level of E2 ($P> = 0.05$)

- The effect of three treatment groups on the E2 level was not significantly different ($P>0.05$).

5-1-1-4: According to decrease in the level of LH:

- KBW significantly decreased the level of LH ($P<0.05$).
- HT significantly decreased the level of LH ($P<0.05$).
- ACU+KBW didn't make a significant decrease on the Level of LH in patients. ($P>0.05$)

- The effect of three treatment groups on the LH level was not significantly different ($P> 0.05$).

5-1-1-5: According to decrease in the number of symptoms:

- KBW was effective in decreasing the number of symptoms ($P<0.05$).
- ACU+KBW was effective in decreasing the number of symptoms ($p<0.001$).
- HT was effective in decreasing the number of symptoms ($p<0.001$).
- According to one way ANOVA, the effect of three treatment groups on Number of Symptoms was not significantly different ($P>0.05$). [114]

Summery of therapeutic response in main groups:

- KBW is effective in the treatment of MRS by decreasing KI, LH and number of symptoms.
- ACU + KBW is effective in the treatment of MRS by decreasing KI, FSH and number of symptoms.
- HT is effective in the treatment of MRS by decreasing KI, LH and number of symptoms.

- The effect of ACU + KBW is significantly better than KBW in decreasing KI but their effect on FSH, LH, E2 and number of symptoms is similar.
- There isn't any significant difference between the effect of ACU+KBW and HT on KI, FSH, LH, E2 and number of symptoms.
- HT is significantly better than KBW in decreasing FSH but no significant difference on KI, E2, LH and number of symptoms.

5-1-2 The therapeutic response in subgroups (peri menopause patients vs. post menopause patients)

- Peri menopause and post menopause patient's response to KBW and ACU+KBW according to KI, FSH, LH and E2 is not significantly different. Post menopause patients responded to HT significantly better than Perimenopause patients (according to KI).
- Peri menopause patients respond to KBW better than Post menopause patients, however the difference is not significant (according to KI).

- In Perimenopause patients there isn't any significant difference between three treatments' effect on KI; however according to FSH, HT is significantly better than

KBW but similar to ACU+KBW.

- Between three treatments KBW has the weakest effects on post menopause patients; significantly different from ACU+KBW and HT.

5-1-3 correlations between treatment response and patients' symptoms or conditions

First we evaluated the distribution of symptoms before the treatment in three treatment groups by Kruskel- Wallis test to know whether or not there is significant difference between three treatment groups about each symptom. Then the ...test was done on some of the symptoms with equal distribution in treatment groups including Hot flash, Insomnia, Weakness, Palpitation, and Constipation and having 5 zone hot sensations. About 5 zone hot sensations, Chi- square test was used to evaluate the equality of distribution of this symptom in treatment groups. Paresthesia, Nervousness, Depressed mood, Arthralgia, Headache, Formication and Mouth dryness were excluded from the list because of significant difference in their distribution between three treatment groups.

- "Time distance from menopause to the beginning of treatment" in post menopause patients is not a prognostic factor for changes in patients' symptoms by treatment. However our sample size in subgroups of Peimenopause and post menopause patients is not enough to judge.

  About hormonal changes, some correlations have been found. They suggest "TD from menopause to treatment" as a prognostic factor in post menopause patients when we treat the patient with ACU+KBW or HT. Since the relation is direct, it means that in post menopause patients the longer the "TD from menopause to treatment", the better effect on decreasing FSH would be achieved by ACU+KBW or HT. This finding is far from our expectation.
- "Time distance from beginning of menses irregularity to the initiation of treatment" is not a prognostic factor for changes in symptoms by the treatment.

  About hormonal changes, In HT group "time distance from beginning of menses irregularity to the initiation of treatment" could be considered as a prognostic factor for decreasing LH negatively. It means that the more "TD from beginning of menses irregularity to the initiation of treatment" the less decrease in LH would be achieved by HT.
- Severity of **hot flash** could be considered as a prognostic factor which negatively predicts the patient's response (decreasing KI) to KBW, HT and totally to the treatment. This finding is more definite and reliable when we consider all of the treatments as a whole not in treatment groups ($p<0.001$). It means that the more severe hot flash before the treatment patient has, the less therapeutic effect on symptoms will be achieved.
- Severity of **insomnia** could be considered as a prognostic factor which negatively predicts the patient's response (decreasing KI) to ACU+KBW and totally to the treatment. It means that the more severe insomnia before the treatment patient has, the less therapeutic effect on symptoms will be achieved by ACU+KBW and totally by treatment.

Besides, there were correlations between severity of insomnia and FSH level (negative) totally and LH level (direct) in HT group.

- Severity of **weakness** could be considered as a prognostic factor which negatively predicts the patient's response (decreasing KI) to the treatment totally. It means that the more severe weakness before the treatment patient has, the less therapeutic effect on symptoms will be achieved by the treatment totally.
- Severity of **palpitation** could be a prognostic factor which negatively predicts the patient's response (decreasing KI) to ACU+KBW and to the treatment totally. It means that the more severe palpitation before the treatment patient has, the less therapeutic effect on symptoms will be achieved by ACU+KBW and the treatment totally. This correlation is strong ($p<0.001$)
- Having **5 zones hot sensation** before the treatment would be a predictor of good prognosis for the treatment of symptoms by KBW.
- According to our findings, severity of **constipation** before treatment had negative correlations with increase in E2 and decrease in LH by ACU+KBW and increase in E2 totally by treatment.

Summery of Correlations:

- The severity of **hot flash**, Insomnia, weakness, **palpitation** and having "**5 zone hot sensations**" before the treatment would be a prognostic factor for changes in symptoms by the treatment.
- Severity of Hot Flash before the treatment may indicate poor prognosis by KBW and HT. Having 5 zone hot sensations before the treatment predicts a good prognosis by KBW.
- Factors whose severity before the treatment indicates poor prognosis by ACU+ KBW include insomnia and palpitation.

5-2 Assessment of similarities and differences with other studies

Back to the Review of literature, there was a study conducted by Wang Lei and colleagues. Although in this study, **KBW** was used as the control group (Mei shen granules as the main group), but we can use the effective rate of KBW from this study. One of the inclusion criteria of this study is similar to our study: Perimenopausal women with **syndrome** of Kidney Yin Deficiency including patients with deficiency of Liver and Kidney or Disharmony between Heart and Kidney. About the first outcome which is "total effective rate", we don't know what the definition and scale is for effectivity in this article. Any way the total effective rate for Kun Bao Wan group is 86.6% in this article vs. 43.64% in our study. The total effective rate in our study is the average of difference between Kuppermann Index before and after the treatment. In their study there was an increase in serum level of E2, compared with before treatment in both KBW group and

Mei shen granule group (P <0.001). This is in contrast with our study in which KBW didn't make any significant increase in the level of E2 (P> = 0.05). Also they found that FSH and LH declined in different degrees comparing with before treatment (P <0. 05, P <0.001). Our study doesn't confirm their results about FSH since we found KBW didn't make a significant decrease on the Level of FSH in patients. (P>0.05) but confirms their findings about LH. We also found that KBW significantly decreased the level of LH (P<0.05).

In another study by geng jia wei the effect of 3 months treatment by "Geng An tang" was compared with "Kun Bao Wan" as the control group in women with menopausal symptoms. Like the previous study, KBW was used as the control group in this study, but we can use the effective rate of KBW from this study which was 70.8% in KBW group; while in our study the KI difference was 43.64%. Again in this article the definition and scale of effectivity is not mentioned clearly. In fact the information from this study is not enough to judge or compare.

Our study confirms the results of studies who found **acupuncture** effective in the treatment of VMS:

Avis and colleagues showed that there was a significant decrease in mean frequency of hot flashes between weeks 1 and 8 across all groups.

Xia and colleagues in their study compared EA and Hormone therapy in the treatment of MRS. They found that Kupperman index of EA group decreased significantly (P < 0.01). Our study confirms this result because in our study ACU+KBW significantly decreased Kuperman Index too. In their study, FSH and LH of EA group decreased significantly (P < 0.01). Our study confirms the decrease of FSH by Acupuncture but not LH. In our study, ACU+KBW didn't make a significant decrease on the Level of LH in patients (P>0.05). In their study, serum E2 of EA and medication groups increased significantly (P < 0. 01). Our study doesn't confirm this results since in our study, ACU + KBW and HT didn't make any significant increase in the level of E2 (P> = 0.05). In their study, Serum LH and E2 levels of EA group were significantly lower than those of medication group (P < 0.05); while in contrast to that, our study shows that the effect of ACU+KBW and HT on the level of E2 and LH were not significantly different (P>0.05). In their study no significant difference was found between two groups in Kupperman index. Our study confirms this fact since in our study there isn't any significant difference between the effect of ACU+KBW and HT too.

In a similar study to the former mentioned, Qin and colleagues showed that serum FSH and LH contents decreased significantly and serum E2 increased considerably (P < 0.001) compared with its basic values. Our study confirms their results about FSH but not about E2 and LH since there was no significant increase in E2 and no significant decrease in LH by ACU+KBW in our research. The same conclusion comes with comparison between our study and the study by Jin and colleagues in 2007.

Our study confirms the results of study by Wyon and colleagues in 2004 that compared 2 groups of acupuncture with Hormone therapy and found that the Kupperman index decreased ($p < 0.001$).

In brief, this study is in accordance with studies that found acupuncture effective in releasing symptoms of MRS.

5-3 advantages and shortcomings of this study

This study introduces some prognostic factors which is a new idea in decision making for women with MRS. The results of this study are promising for the effect of Acupuncture and herbal medicine, since the effect of these two traditional therapies are as well as the conventional hormone therapy according to our study.
Talking about some shortcomings, our sample size was not enough to judge about some findings in subgroups. Also, we didn't have a control group without any treatment to differentiate the decrease in symptoms due to a natural process or due to our treatment. Furthermore, we didn't have a group of Sham acupuncture to give a more valid idea about the effects of acupuncture and differentiate the real effect of acupuncture from placebo.

5-4 Suggestions for future studies

We suggest running a study with 3 control groups: a group of hormone therapy, a group of sham acupuncture, and a group without any therapy besides the herbal medicine group and acupuncture group; to increase the reliability of results and see whether or not acupuncture is really better than sham acupuncture; and whether or not herbal medicine is effective in comparison with women who doesn't receive any treatment. In this way, the placebo effect of herbs or acupuncture will be diminished and judgment would be more reliable. Up to now, literature is still doubtful about this issue.

Chapter Six

Conclusion

Our study revealed that the herbal medicine we used (KBW) and acupuncture as two Traditional Chinese Medicine treatments both are significantly effective in decreasing the symptoms of women with MRS; even acupuncture + KBW is as effective as the conventional hormone therapy in decreasing the symptoms also about the hormonal changes after therapy. According to our results, the effect of ACU + KBW is significantly better than KBW in relieving symptoms but their effect on FSH, LH and E2 is similar. KBW was not as well as HT and ACU+KBW in decreasing symptoms. HT was significantly better than KBW in decreasing FSH but no significant difference on KI, E2 and LH. [114]

Also we compared the therapeutic response between perimenopause and post menopause patients. Peri menopause and post menopause patient's response to KBW and ACU+KBW was not significantly different but Post menopause patients responded to HT significantly better than Perimenopause patients (according to KI).
Between three treatments, KBW has the weakest effects on post menopause patients; significantly different from ACU+KBW and HT. In Perimenopause patients there wasn't any significant difference between three treatments' effects on KI.

Finally we found some correlations between severity of some symptoms and response to treatment which led to introducing some prognostic factors in the treatment of MRS. The severity of hot flash, Insomnia, weakness, palpitation and having "5 zone hot sensations" before the treatment would be prognostic factors for changes in symptoms by the treatment.

7
References

[1]- NIH state-of-the-science conference statement on management of menopause-related symptoms. NIH Consens State Sci Statements. 2005; 22(1):5-14.

[2]- AACE Menopause Guidelines Revision Task Force. American Association of Clinical Endocrinologists medical guidelines for clinical practice for the diagnosis and treatment of menopause. Endocr Pract. 2006;12:315-37.

[3]- North American Menopause Society. Estrogen and progestogen use in peri- and postmenopausal women: March 2007 position statement of The North American Menopause Society. Menopause. 2007;14:168-82.

[4]-Elena M. umland, Treatment Strategies for Reducing the Burden of Menopause-Associated Vasomotor Symptoms. JMCP, 2008, 14(3), pp 4-19.

[5]- Ryan J, et al. A prospective study of the association between endogenous hormones and depressive symptoms in postmenopausal women. *Menopause* 2009 Jan 21.

[6]- Utian WH. Psychosocial and socioeconomic burden of vasomotor symptoms in menopause: a comprehensive review. Health Qual Life Outcomes. 2005;3:47

[7]- McVeigh C: Perimenopause: more than hot flushes and night sweats for some Australian women. J Obstet Gynecol Neonatal Nurs 2005, 34:21-27.

[8]- Williams RE et al, Menopause-specific questionnaire assessment in US population-based study shows negative impact on health-related quality of life. Maturitas. 2009 Jan 19. [Epub ahead of print]

[9]- Williams RE, et al. Health care seeking and treatment for menopausal symptoms in the United States. Maturitas. 2007;58:348-58

[10]- North American Menopause Society. Treatment of menopause-associated vasomotor symptoms: position statement of The North American Menopause Society. Menopause. 2004;11:11-33

[11]- Mohyi D, Tabassi K, Simon J: Differential diagnosis of hot flashes. Maturitas 1997, 27:203-214.

[12]- U.S. Census Bureau. Annual estimates of the population by five-year age groups and sex for the United States: April 1, 2000 to July 1, 2006. Available at: www.census.gov/popest/national/asrh/NC-EST2006/NC-EST2006-01.xls.
Accessed December 9, 2007.

[13]- Botteman MF, Shah NP, Lian J, Pashos CL, Simon JA. A cost-effectiveness evaluation of two continuous-combined hormone therapies for the management of moderate-to-severe vasomotor symptoms. Menopause. 2004;11:343-55.

[14]- Lomax P and Schonbaum E. Postmenopausal hot flushes and their management. *Pharmacol Ther* 1993;57:347-58

[15]- Casper RF, Yen SS. Neuroendocrinology of menopausal flushes: a hypothesis of flush mechanism. Clin Endocrinol (Oxf) 1985;22:293-312

[16]- Schurz B, et al. Beta endorphin levels during the climacteric period. Maturitas 1988;10:45-50

[17]- Cagnacci A, et al. Neuroendocrine and clinical effects of transdermal 17 beta-estradiol in postmenopausal women. Maturitas 1991;13:283-96

[18]- Leslie RD, et al. Sensitivity to enkephalin as a cause of non-insulin dependent diabetes. Lancet 1979;1:341-3

[19]- Berendsen HH. The role of Serotonin in hot flushes. Maturitas 2000;36:155-64
[20]- Gonzales GF, Carrilo C. Blood serotonin levels in postmenopausal women: effect of age and serum oestradiol levels. Maturitas 1993;17:23-9
[21]- Blum I, et al. The effect of estrogen replacement therapy on plasma serotonin and catecholamines of postmenopausal women. Isr J Med Sci 1996;32:1158-62
[22]- Freedman RR, Krell W. Reduced thermoregulatory null zone in post menopausal women with hot f lashes. Am J Obstet Gynecol. 1999; 181:66-70.
[23]- Utian WH. Biosynthesis and physiologic effects of estrogen and pathophysiologic effects of estrogen deficiency: a review. Am J Obstet Gynecol. 1989;161:1828-31
[24]- MacKay HT. Gynecology. In: Tierney LM, McPhee SJ, Papadakis MA, ed. Current Medical Diagnosis & Treatment. San Francisco, CA: Lange Medical Books/McGraw-Hill; 2004:726.
[25]- Crandall CJ, Crawford SL, Gold EB. Vasomotor symptom prevalence is associated with polymorphisms in sex steroid-metabolizing enzymes and receptors. Am J Med. 2006;119(9 suppl 1):S52-S60.
[26]- Mitrunen K, Hirvonen A. Molecular epidemiology of sporadic breast cancer: the role of polymorphic genes involved in oestrogen biosynthesis and metabolism. Mutat Res. 2003;54:9-41.
[27]- Gruber CJ, Tschugguel W, Schneeberger C, Huber JC. Production and actions of estrogens. N Engl J Med. 2002;346:340-52.s
[28]- Burger H.G. and Dennerstein L. Cycle and hormone changes during perimenopause: the key role of ovarian function. *Menopause* 2008. 15(4): 603-612
[29]- Griffiths F. Women's control and choice regarding HRT. Soc Sci Med ,1999;49:469-81
[30]- Hulley S, Grady D, Bush T, Furberg C,Herrington D, Riggs B, et al. Randomized trial of estrogen plus progestin for secondary prevention of coronary heart disease in postmenopausal women. JAMA 1998;280:605-13
[31]- Writing Group for the Women's Health Initiative Investigators. Risks and benefits of estrogen plus progesterone in healthy post-menopausal women. JAMA 2002;288:321-33
[32]- Abraham S, Perz J, Clarkson R, Llewellyn-Jones D. Australian women's perceptions of hormone replacement therapy over 10 years. Maturitas 1995;21:91-5
[33]- Rymer J, Morris EP. Extracts from Clinical Evidence: menopausal symptoms. BMJ 2002;321:1516-9
[34]- Eriksen PS, Rasmussen H. Low dose 17â oestradiol vaginal tablets in the treatment of atrophic vaginities: a double blind placebo controlled study. Eur J Obstet Gynaecol Reprod Biol, 1992;44:137-44
[35]- Zethraeus N, Johannesson M, Henricksson P, Strand RT. The impact of hormone replacement therapy on quality of life and willingness to pay. Br J Obstet Gynaecol 1999;104:1191-5
[36]- Cooper C. Epidemiology and definition of osteoporosis. In: Compston JE, ed. Osteoporosis: new perspectives on causes, prevention and treatment. London: Royal College of Physicians, 1996:1-10

[37]- Torgerson DJ, Bell-Syer SE. Hormone replacement therapy and prevention of non-vertebral fractures: a meta-analysis of randomised trials. JAMA 2001;285:2891-7

[38]- Grodstein F, et al. Postmenopausal hormone therapy and the risk of colorectal cancer: a review and meta-analysis. Am J Med 1999;106:574-82

[39]- Rymer J et al, Making decisions about hormone replacement therapy, BMJ 2003, 326, pp322-326

[40]- Grodstein F, Stampfer M. The epidemiology of coronary heart disease and estrogen replacement in postmenopausal women. Prog Cardiovasc Dis 1995;38:199-210

[41]- Grady D, Gebretsadick T, Kerlikowske K, Ernster V, Petitti D. Hormone replacement therapy and endometrial cancer risk: a meta-analysis. Obstet Gynaecol 1995;85:304-13

[42]- Hulley S, Furberg C, Barret-Connore C, Cauley J, Grady D, Haskell W, et al. Non-cardiovascular disease outcomes during 6.8 years on hormone therapy: heart and estrogen/progestin replacement study follow up (HERS II). JAMA 2002;288:58-66

[43]- Daly E, Vessey MP, Hawkins MM, Carson JL, Gough P, Marsh S. Risk of venous thromboembolism in users of HRT. Lancet 1996;348:977-80

[44]- Jick H, Derby LE, Myers MW, Vasilakis C, Newton KM. Risk of hospital admission for idiopathic venous thromboembolism among users of postmenopausal oestrogens. Lancet 1996;348:981-3

[45]- Grady D,Wenger NK,Herrington D,Khan S, Furberg C,Hunninghake D, et al. Postmenopausal hormone replacement therapy increases risk for venous thromboembolism disease: the heart and estrogen/progestin replacement study. Ann Intern Med 2000;132:689-96

[46]- Hunter MS, O'Dea I. Perception of future health risks in mid-aged women: estimates with and without behavioural changes and hormone replacement therapy. Maturitas 1999;33:37-43.

[47]- Beresford S,Weiss NS, Voigt LF,McKnight B. Risk of endometrial cancer in relation to use of oestrogen combined with cyclic progestogen therapy in postmenopausal women. Lancet 1997;349:458-61.

[48]- Weiderpass E, Adami HO, Baron JA, Magnusson C, Bergstrom R, Lindgren A, et al. Risk of endometrial cancer following estrogen replacement with and without progestins. J Natl Cancer Inst 1999;91:1131-7

[49]- Sturdee DW, Ulrich LG, Barlow DH,Wells M, Campbell MJ, Vessey MP, et al. The endometrial response to sequential and continuous combined oestrogen/progestogen replacement therapy. Br J Obstet Gynaecol 2000;107:1392-400

[50]- Wells M, et al. Effect on endometrium of long term treatment with continuous combined estrogen-progestogen replacement therapy: follow up study. BMJ 2002;325:239

[51]- Lacey JV, et al. Menopausal hormone replacement therapy and risk of ovarian cancer. JAMA 2002;288:334-41

[52]- Sturdee DW. The menopausal hot flush--anything new? Maturitas. 2008 May 20;60(1):42-9.

[53]- Kupferer EM et al, Complementary and alternative medicine use for vasomotor symptoms among women who have discontinued hormone therapy. J Obstet Gynecol Neonatal Nurs. 2009 Jan-Feb;38(1):50-9.
[54]- Innes KE, et al. Menopause, the metabolic syndrome, and mind-body therapies. Menopause. 2008 Sep-Oct;15(5):1005-13.
[55]- Lee MS, et al. Yoga for menopausal symptoms: a systematic review. Menopause. 2009 May-Jun;16(3):602-8
[56]- Gold EB et al, Cross-sectional analysis of specific complementary and alternative medicine (CAM) use by racial/ethnic group and menopausal status: the Study of Women's Health Across the Nation (SWAN). *Menopause*. 2007 Jul-Aug;14(4):601-5.
[57]- Rees M. Alternative treatments for the menopause. Best Pract Res Clin Obstet Gynaecol. 2009 Feb;23(1):151-61.
[58]- Giovanni Maciocia. Obstetrics and Gynecology in Chinese Medicine. Churchill Livingstone, New York, New York, U.S.A., 1998:741-763) (Tan Yong, et al. Gynecology of Traditional Chinese Medicine. People's Medical Publishing House. Beijing, 2007: 304-308
[59]- West Z. Acupuncture within the National Health Service: a personal perspective. *Complement Ther Nurs Midwifery* 1997;3:83-6
[60]- Han JS. Acupuncture: neuropeptide release produced by electrical stimulation of different frequencies. *Trends Neurosci* 2003;26:17-22
[61]- Shen J. Research on the neurophysiological mechanisms of acupuncture: review of selected studies and methodological issues. *J Altern Complement Med* 2001;7(Suppl 1): s121-7
[62]- Cabyoglu, et al. The mechanism of acupuncture and clinical applications. Int J Neurosci. 2006 Feb;116(2):115-25
[63]- Omura Y. Pathophysiology of acupuncture on cardiovascular and nervous systems. *Acupunct Electro-Therapeutics Res* 1975;1:55-141.
[64]- Filshie J, Bolton T, Browne D, Ashley S. Acupuncture and self acupuncture for long-term treatment of vasomotor symptoms in cancer patients - audit and treatment algorithm. *Acu-punct Med* 2005;23:171-80
[65]- Roelofs J, et al. Expectations of an-algesia do not affect spinal nociceptive R-III reflex activity: an experimental study into the mechanism of placebo-induced analgesia. *Pain* 2000;89:75-80
[66]- Johansen O, Brox J, Flaten MA. Placebo and nocebo responses, cortisol, and circulating beta-endorphin. *Psychosom Med* 2003;65:768-90
[67]- Ernst E, White A. Life-threatening adverse reactions after acupuncture? A systematic re-view. *Pain* 1997;71:123-6
[68]- Melchart D, Weidenhammer W, Streng A, et al. Prospective investigation of adverse effects of acupuncture in 97 733 patients. *Arch Intern Med* 2004;164:104-5
[69]- White A, Hayhoe S, Hart A, Ernst E. Adverse events following acupuncture: prospective sur-vey of 32 000 consultations with doctors and physiotherapists. *Br Med J* 2001;323:485-6
[70]- Collaborative Group on Hormonal Factors in Breast Cancer. Breast cancer and hormone replacement therapy: collaborative reanalysis of data

from 51 epidemiological studies of 52,705 women with breast cancer and 108,411 women without breast cancer. *Lancet* 1997; 350:1047-59

[71]- Hormone replacement therapy and venous thromboembolism. Royal College of Obstetri-cians and Gynaecologists. Top guideline no. 19. Revised January 2004

[72]- Curb JD, Prentice RL, Bray PF, et al. Venous thrombosis and conjugated equine estrogen in women without a uterus. *Arch I ntern Med* 2006;166:772-80

[73]- Wang Lei, et al. Meishen granules treated 30 cases of menopausal syndromes. New Journal of Traditional Chinese Medicine 2008;40(10),pp 59-60

[74]- geng jia wei.Geng An Tang treated the menopause syndrome in 96 cases. Zhong guo lin chuang yi sheng, 2002, May;50, p 46

[75]- Yan Hua, kun bao wan treat manopuse sysptoms for 36 cases. Zhong guo ming jian liao fa 2006 October;14:38-39

[76]- An Rui Xian, 1 case report of Urticaria by kun bao wan. Xin yi xue zazhi 2008;39:202

[77]- Xu Jian. Set up a quality standard of Kun Bao Wan. Journal of Chang Chun, 2006;22:47-48

[78]- Lee MS, et al. Acupuncture for treating menopausal hot flushes: a systematic review. Climacteric 2009 Feb;12(1):16-25.

[79]- Alfhaily F. and Ewies A. A. A.. Acupuncture in managing menopausal symptoms: hope or mirage?.*Climacteric* 2007;10:371-80

[80]- Kronenberg F. and Fugh-Berman A. Complementary and alternative medicine for menopausal symptoms: a review of randomized, controlled trials. *Ann Intern Med* 2002.19;137(10):805-13

[81]- Avis NE, et al. A randomized, controlled pilot study of acupuncture treatment for menopausal hot flashes. *Menopause*. 2008 Nov-Dec;15(6):1070-8.

[82]- Xia XH, et al. Multicentral randomized controlled clinical trials about treatment of perimenopausal syndrome with electroacupuncture of sanyinjiao (SP 6). *Zhen Ci Yan Jiu*. 2008 Aug;33(4):262-6

[83]- Qin, et al. Effects of electroacupuncture of Sanyinjiao (SP 6) on genito-endocrine in patients with perimenopausal syndrome. *Zhen Ci Yan Jiu*. 2007 Aug;32(4):255-9

[84]- Jin H, et al. Clinical observation on acupuncture at the five-zangshu for treatment of perimenopausal syndrome. Zhongguo Zhen Jiu. 2007 Aug;27(8):572-4

[85]- Vincent A, et al. Acupuncture for hot flashes: a randomized, sham-controlled clinical study. Menopause. 2007 Jan-Feb;14(1):45-52

[86]- Zaborowska E, et al. Effects of acupuncture, applied relaxation, estrogns and placebo on hot flushes in post menopausal women: an analysis of two prospective, parallel, randomized studies. *Climacteric* 2007;10:38-45

[87]- Ma XP, et al. Effects of acupuncture on granulocyte apoptosis and expressions of apoptosis-associated genes in the ovary of perimenopausal rats. Zhongguo Zhen Jiu. 2007 May;27(5):357-61

[88]- Huang MI, et al. A randomized controlled pilot study of acupuncture for postmenopausal hot flashes: effect on nocturnal hot flashes and sleep quality. *Fertil Steril* 2006;86:700-10

[89]- Wyon Y, et al. A comparison of acupuncture and oral estradiol treatment of vasomotor symptoms in postmenopausal women. *Climacteric* 2004; 7:153-64

[90]- Cohen SM, Rousseau ME, Carey BL. Can acupuncture ease the symptoms of menopause? *Holist Tlurs Pract* 2003;17:295-9

[91]- Dong H, Ludicke F, Comte I, Campana A, Graff P, Bischof P. An exploratory pilot study of acupuncture on the quality of life and reproduc tive hormone secretion in menopausal women. *J Altern Complement Med* 2001;7:651-8

[92]- Grille M, et al. L'emploi therapeutique de l'acupuncture dans la menopause. (Experiennces de l'hopital de Ravenne et de Bologne). *La Revue Francaise de Medecine Traditionelle Chinoise* 1989;133: 65-6

[93]- Conchetto D. Orientation diagnostigue et ther-apeutigue dans le syndrome climaterique en medicine chinoise. *La Revue Francaise de Medecine Traditionell chinoise* 1989;133:55-6

[94]- Limarti L, Ricciarelli E. Utilisation des points dorsaux paravertebraaux dans les syndromes anxio-depressifs climateriques. *La Revue Fran-caise de Medecine Traditionelle Chinoise* 1989;133:70-1

[95]- Sotte L. Therapies des syndromes polyarticu-laires en menopause. *La Revue Francaise de Medecine Traditionelle Chinoise* 1989;133:57-9

[96]- Frisk J, et al. Long-term follow-up of acupuncture and hormone therapy on hot flushes in women with breast cancer: a prospective, randomized, controlled multicenter trial. Climacteric. 2008 Apr;11(2):166-74

[97]- Nedstrand E, Wijma K, Wyon Y, Hammar M. Vasomotor symptoms decrease in women with breast cancer randomized to treatment with applied relaxation or electro-acupuncture: a preliminary study. *Climacteric* 2005;8:243-50

[98]- Porzio G, Trapasso T, Martelli S, et al. Acupuncture in the treatment of menopause-related symptoms in women taking tamoxifen. *Tumori* 2002; 8 8:12 8-30

[99]- Tukmachi E. Treatment of hot flushes in breast cancer patients with acupuncture. *Acupuncture Med* 2000;18:22-7

[100]- Cumins SM, Murray Brant A. Does acupuncture influence the vasomotor symptoms experienced by breast cancer patients taking tamoxifen? *Acupunct Med* 2000;18:28

[101]- Towlerton G, Filshie J, O'Brien M, Duncan A. Acupuncture in the control of vasomotor symp-toms caused by tamoxifen. Palliat *Med* 1999;13:445

[102]- Andrikoula M, Prelevic G. Menopausal hot flushes revisited. Climacteric. 2009 Feb;12(1):3-15

[103]- No authors listed. Herbal medicines for menopausal symptoms. Drug Ther Bull. 2009 Jan;47(1):2-6.

[104]- Bair YA, et al. Use of complementary and alternative medicine during the menopause transition: longitudinal results from the Study of Women's Health Across the Nation. Menopause. 2008 Jan-Feb;15(1):32-43.

[105]- Keenan NL et al, Severity of menopausal symptoms and use of both conventional and complementary/alternative therapies. Menopause. 2003 Nov-Dec;10(6):491-3.

[106]- Nelson HD, et al. Nonhormonal therapies for menopausal hot flashes: systematic review and meta-analysis. JAMA. 2006 May 3;295(17):2057-71.
[107]- van der Sluijs CP, et al. A randomized placebo-controlled trial on the effectiveness of an herbal formula to alleviate menopausal vasomotor symptoms. Menopause. 2008 Dec 4.
[108]- Haines CJ, et al. A randomized, double-blind, placebo-controlled study of the effect of a Chinese herbal medicine preparation (Dang Gui Buxue Tang) on menopausal symptoms in Hong Kong Chinese women. Climacteric. 2008 Jun;11(3):244-51.
[109]- Green J, et al. Treatment of menopausal symptoms by qualified herbal practitioners: a prospective, randomized controlled trial. Fam Pract. 2007 Oct;24(5):468-74.
[110]- Palacio C, et al. Black cohosh for the management of menopausal symptoms : a systematic review of clinical trials. Drugs Aging. 2009;26(1):23-36.
[111]- Newton KM, Treatment of vasomotor symptoms of menopause with black cohosh, multibotanicals, soy, hormone therapy, or placebo: a randomized trial. Ann Intern Med. 2006 Dec 19;145(12):869-79.
[112]- Lethaby AE, et al. Phytoestrogens for vasomotor menopausal symptoms. Cochrane Database Syst Rev. 2007 Oct 17;(4):CD001395.
[113]- Adaikan PG, et al. Efficacy of red clover isoflavones in the menopausal rabbit model. Fertil Steril. 2008 Oct 28.

[114]- Azizi H, Feng Liu Y, Du L, Hua Wang C, Bahrami-Taghanaki H, Ollah Esmaily H, Azizi H, Ou Xue X. Menopause-related symptoms: traditional Chinese medicine vs hormone therapy. Altern Ther Health Med. 2011 Jul-Aug;17(4):48-53.

8 Acknowledgements

Acknowledgement

I am heartily thankful to my supervisor, Professor Xiao Ou Xue, whose encouragement, guidance and immense support from the initial to the final level enabled me to develop an understanding of the subject and overcoming the difficulties in the process of research.

Besides my supervisor, I would like to express my gratitude to the rest of my thesis committee: Dr. Yan Feng Liu, Dr. Lin Du, Dr. Chao Hua Wang and Dr. Habib Esmaily for their great help, encouragement and insightful comments. Dr. Yan Feng Liu taught Chinese Medicine Gynecology to me and kindly accepted me in her clinic to collect my thesis data. I had this chance to study and practice in her clinic for around two years which was really a worth period. She has provided assistance to me in numerous ways. Dr. Du helpfully and generously did the acupuncture for my patients free of charge. Also she gave me the chance to learn and practice acupuncture in her clinic and lent me a hand whenever I need. Dr. Wang sincerely accepted me in her clinic for collecting my research cases, solved the problems with her tact, guided and supported me humbly. Dr. Esmaily, the Iranian professor of Statistics not only helped me to analyze the data of this research patiently but also taught me a lot.

I would like to thank all of the doctors in Gynecology clinic of Dongzhimen Hospital for their kindly help by introducing patients to me; nurses of Gynecology clinic and ward of Dongzhimen Hospital and Peking University People Hospital, laboratory of Dongzhimen Hospital for their sincere aid and also my dear patients for their cooperation with me.

I am grateful to my Chinese friends and classmates who always helped me in defeating the numerous difficulties of learning in Chinese language; especially my gratitude goes to my friends Xiao Yan Dou, Yun Zhi Chen and Lu Liu who honestly assisted me by my thesis.

I offer my regards and blessings to all of those who supported me in any respect during the completion of the project.

Lastly, I want to express my gratitude to my family; my sisters and my brother for their reassurance, inspiration and helps.

I dedicate my thesis to my dear father and mother whose deep inspiration supported me all the time and every thing I have belong to them.

Hoda Azizi

致 谢

衷心感谢我的导师薛晓鸥教授！导师对我的指导、鼓励和由始至终的巨大支持，使我能够克服研究过程中的一切困难，最终完成此项临床研究。

此外，感谢论文组的其他成员，给了我很大的帮助、鼓励和启发，他们是：刘雁峰教授，杜琳教授，王朝华教授以及 Habib Esmaily 教授。刘雁峰教授指导我学习中医妇科，允许我在她的诊室收集论文数据。在她的诊室学习和实践这两年的时间，给了我各方面的帮助，使我获益匪浅。杜琳教授为我的病人做免费的针刺治疗，使我有机会在她的诊室学习和实践针灸学，带给我极大的帮助。王吵华教授允许我在她的诊室收集临床病例，用她的经验给我许多指导和支持。伊朗统计学教授 Dr. Esmaily，帮助我分析此项研究的数据，并教给我很多知识。

感谢东直门医院妇科所有的医生，她们无私地把病人介绍给我；感谢东直门医院和北京大学人民医院的妇科护士，东直门医院实验室的老师给我真诚的帮助，以及我的病人对我的研究的充分配合。

感谢我所有的中国朋友和同学，帮助我战胜学习中文上的很多困难。特别感谢我的朋友窦晓燕，陈云芝和刘璐在写论文中给我坦诚的帮助。

在此项研究完成之际，我衷心地感谢和祝福所有给我各方面支持的人。

最后，感谢我的家人，我的兄弟姐妹给我的信心、激励和帮助。我把我的论文献给我亲爱的父亲母亲，他们一直以来给我深深的鼓励，我获得的一切成绩都是属于他们的。

Hoda Azizi

9
Appendix

9-1 Algorithm

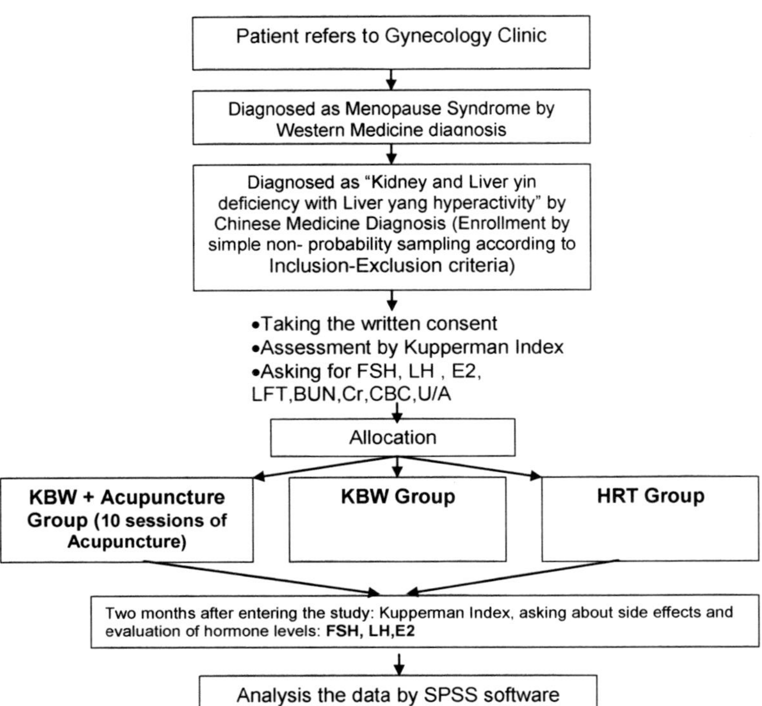

9-2 Questionnaire

调查问卷

治疗组:

中药治疗组(坤宝丸): ( ) 针灸 +坤宝丸: ( ) 激素替代治疗组: ( )

姓名: ______________ **年龄:** (______________)

已婚( ) 未婚( )

学历: （ ）小学程度以下，（ ）小学，（ ）初中，（ ）中专，（ ）高中，（ ）专科/高职，（ ）本科，（ ）研究生，（ ）博士及以上

联系电话:______________(手机) ___________(住宅) __________(办公室)

地址: ____

既往史: （ ）有乳癌病史或不明原因的乳房肿块 （ ）子宫内膜癌 （ ）血栓性疾病 （ ）不明原因的阴道出血 （ ）未经治疗的高血压 （ ）肝病 （ ）肾病

（ ）其他并:

____

用药史: ____

最近三次月经日期: LMP(__________) 2LMP(__________) 3LMP(__________)

开始月经紊乱日起: (______________)

手术引起的绝经: （ ）是 （ ）不是

手术史: ____

实验数据:

	实验日期	数据
研究前		**FSH (** **)** **LH (** **)** **E2 (** **)**
8 周后		**FSH (** **)** **LH (** **)** **E2 (** **)**

初诊日期: (______________)

Kupperman 量表包括的症状

1、**潮热出汗**

（ ）无

（ ）

（ ）<3 次/天 （ ）

（ ）3-9 次/天 （ ）

（ ）＞10 次/天 （ ）

2、感觉异常

（ ）无 （ ）

（ ）有时 （ ）

（ ）经常有刺痛、麻木、耳鸣等 （ ）

（ ）经常而且严重 （ ）

3、失眠

（ ）无 （ ）

（ ）有时 （ ）

（ ）经常 （ ）

（ ）经常且严重需服安定类药 （ ）

4、焦躁

（ ）无 （ ）

（ ）有时 （ ）

（ ）经常 （ ）

（ ）经常不能自控 （ ）

5、忧郁

（ ）无 （ ）

（ ）有时 （ ）

（ ）经常，能自控 （ ）

（ ）失去生活信心 （ ）

6、眩晕

（ ）无 （ ）

（ ）有时 （ ）

（ ）经常，不影响生活 （ ）

（ ）影响生活与工作 （ ）

7、疲倦乏力

（ ）无 （ ）

（ ）有时 （ ）

（ ）经常 （ ）

（ ）日常生活受限 （ ）

8、肌肉骨关节痛

（ ）无 （ ）

（ ）有时 （ ）

（ ）经常，不影响功能 （ ）

（ ）功能障碍 （ ）

9、头痛

（ ）无 （ ）

（ ）有时 （ ）

（ ）经常，能忍受 （ ）
（ ）需服药 （ ）

10、**心悸**

（ ）无 （ ）
（ ）有时 （ ）
（ ）经常，不影响工作 （ ）
（ ）需治疗 （ ）

11、**皮肤蚁走感**

（ ）无 （ ）
（ ）有时 （ ）
（ ）经常，能忍受 （ ）
（ ）需治疗 （ ）

中医诊断标准

1、月经紊乱

（ ）已经停经了 停经日期:________________
（ ）经期延长
（ ）
（ ）经期缩短
（ ）
（ ）经量增多
（ ）
（ ）经量减少
（ ）
（ ）经色鲜红
（ ）

2、烘热汗出: （ ） （ ）
3、五心烦热: （ ） （ ）
4、头目眩晕: （ ） （ ）
5、耳鸣: （ ） （ ）
6、腰膝酸疼: （ ） （ ）
7、足跟疼痛: （ ） （ ）
8、皮肤干燥、瘙痒: （ ） （ ）
9、口干: （ ） （ ）
10、尿少色黄: （ ） （ ）
11、大便干燥: （ ） （ ）
12、眼睛干涩: （ ） （ ）
13、阴道干: （ ） （ ）

14、舌红少苔： （　　　　　）　　（　　　　　）
15、脉细数： （　　　　　）　　（　　　　　）
16、失眠： （　　　　　）　　（　　　　　）
17、心悸： （　　　　　）　　（　　　　　）
18、平时怕冷还是怕热？ （　　　　　）
（　　　　　）
19. 证性： （　　　　　）　　（　　　　　）

患 者 知 情 同 意 书

尊敬的志愿受试者：

您的主治医师拟邀请您参加一项医疗研究。本研究方案在国际通行的有关临床试验研究规范的指导下制定，是安全和合乎医德的，已得到本研究负责单位伦理委员会的批准。

本研究分 3 个组同时进行，共计将有 200 余名患者参加。所有的肾阴虚型更年期患者分为三个治疗组，分别给予坤宝丸(KBW)、坤宝丸加针灸(KBW+Acupuncture)、和激素替代治疗(HRT)。每位患者将按照就诊顺序被随机分配到其中任意一组，应用相应的方法治疗。每位患者的治疗周期为 3 个月，给药前、后要各查一次血、尿、便常规，肝、肾功能、FSH、LH、E_2 等临床研究方案所要求的项目。患者治疗后最后一次相关检查的费用是免费的。

为了评价试验用药的疗效和安全性，有必要在研究期间不再使用其他治疗围绝经期的药物和疗法。

绝大多数患者将从本研究中受益，并且，您将获得一次免费针灸治疗更年期综合征的机会；并且在本研究期间，获得某些全新重要的信息，您的医生将会随时通知您，您有权在任何时间询问有关本研究的任何问题，并且您有权决定在任何时间退出本研究。患者无论何种情况下退出，均必须告诉您的主管医师。不论您是否决定参加本研究，都不会影响您和医生之间的关系。

尽管到目前为止没有发现该治疗中的不良反应，但是任何病情新的变化，应当及时通知您的医生。她/他将对其做出处理并监护您的健康状况。无论何种原因，如您退出本项研究，有很多其他的疗法可替代。医生将会尽全力防止由于本研究可能带来的不良影响。

患者的所有资料归研究者所有，研究者保护患者的隐私权，但在有关部门需要时，有使用这些资料的权利。

患者承诺：

我已阅读并了解上述有关本研究的情况。我同意参加此项研究，并保证尽量按照研究要求与临床医师配合完成试验。

患者签名：__________　　　　　　　　________年____月____日

联系电话：

我已详细向患者介绍了整个研究过程，并告知患者在研究过程中的风险和获益情况。

临床医师签名：____________　　　　　　　　　　　　________年____月____日

联系电话：

CPSIA information can be obtained at www.ICGtesting.com
Printed in the USA
LVOW11s0200210415

435414LV00001B/185/P

9 783639 515114